The Spiritual Dimension of Alternative Medicine

The Spiritual Dimension of Alternative Medicine

A Christian Assessment

ERNEST M. VALEA

RESOURCE *Publications* • Eugene, Oregon

THE SPIRITUAL DIMENSION OF ALTERNATIVE MEDICINE
A Christian Assessment

Copyright © 2020 Ernest M. Valea. All rights reserved. Except for brief quotations in critical publications or reviews, no part of this book may be reproduced in any manner without prior written permission from the publisher. Write: Permissions, Wipf and Stock Publishers, 199 W. 8th Ave., Suite 3, Eugene, OR 97401.

Resource Publications
An Imprint of Wipf and Stock Publishers
199 W. 8th Ave., Suite 3
Eugene, OR 97401

www.wipfandstock.com

PAPERBACK ISBN: 978-1-7252-6050-4
HARDCOVER ISBN: 978-1-7252-6049-8
EBOOK ISBN: 978-1-7252-6051-1

Manufactured in the U.S.A.   01/29/20

Contents

Introduction | vii

1. Human Nature According to Christian Teaching | 1
2. Yoga as Therapy and Religion | 9
    - 2.1 Illusion, Ignorance, Karma, and Reincarnation | 9
    - 2.2 Human Nature and Liberation | 12
    - 2.3 How Much Religion is in Yoga? | 13
    - 2.4 Hatha Yoga Practice and its Defining Elements | 16
    - 2.5 Yoga and its Esoteric Powers and Experiences | 19
    - 2.6 Chakra Healing | 21
    - 2.7 Yoga for Christians? | 23
    - 2.8 Reincarnation and Christianity | 24
3. Anthroposophical Medicine (AM) | 27
    - 3.1 The Four Components of Human Nature | 28
    - 3.2 Four Bodies, Seven Planets, and Seven Healing Metals | 32
    - 3.3 The Treatment for Cancer | 34
    - 3.4 The Spiritual Evolution of Humankind | 35
4. Ayurveda | 39
    - 4.1 Ayurvedic Typology | 39
    - 4.2 Diagnosis and Treatment in Ayurveda | 40
    - 4.3 Ayurveda and its Spiritual Teachings | 43
    - 4.4 Other Hindu Practices in Ayurveda | 46
    - 4.5 Ayurveda and Quantum Physics | 49
    - 4.6 Ayurveda and Christianity | 50

5. Reiki | 53
    5.1 The Nature of Reiki Energy | 54
    5.2 Attempted Scientific Explanations | 57
    5.3 The Role of Spiritual Beings in Reiki | 60
    5.4 Reiki and Christianity | 63
    5.5 Addendum. Therapeutic Touch and Macrobiotics | 68

6. Acupuncture and the Principles of Traditional Chinese Medicine | 72
    6.1 A Brief Introduction to Taoism | 72
    6.2 Tai Chi and Qigong | 74
    6.3 Human Anatomy and Physiology in Acupuncture | 76
    6.4 Diagnosis and Treatment in Acupuncture | 79
    6.5 Human Physiology and the Five Fundamental Elements | 82
    6.6 Acupuncture and Christianity | 85

7. Reflexology | 88
    7.1 Physical Reflexology | 89
    7.2 A Large Variety of Reflexology Forms | 91
    7.3 Reflexology as a Way of Channeling Vital Energy | 92
    7.4 From Reflexology to a Hindu View of Human Nature | 95
    7.5 From Reflexology to Tibetan Buddhism | 97
    7.6 Addendum. Iridology | 101

8. Homeopathy | 103
    8.1 Samuel Hahnemann | 104
    8.2 The Preparation of Homeopathic Remedies | 106
    8.3 The Personalization of Treatment | 108
    8.4 Homeopathy and Science | 111
    8.5 The Vital Force | 113
    8.6 The Vital Force and Mesmerism. Homeopathy as Energy Transfer | 116
    8.7 The Vital Force and the Soul | 119
    8.8 Miasms and Original Sin | 121
    8.9 A Personal Encounter with Homeopathy | 123
    8.10 Addendum. The Bach Floral Remedies | 124

9. Alternative Medicine and the Christian View of Health and Healing | 129

Bibliography | 135
Index | 141

Introduction

TWENTY-THREE YEARS AGO I read a book on alternative medicine written by Samuel Pfeifer, a Swiss medical doctor. His book, *Healing At Any Price?*, delves into the spiritual beliefs involved in alternative medicine and raises serious doubts about its appropriateness for Christians. The most important issue to consider, as the title itself suggests, is whether we look for healing at *any price*. In other words, Pfeifer invites us to consider whether we are willing to make *any* effort, try *any* treatment and see *any* healer to find a cure. Unfortunately many Christians respond to this question in the affirmative.

Such an attitude speaks volumes about what we truly believe and our willingness to lead a holy life. Our true beliefs are revealed by what we do, the way we conduct our daily life, and the means we use to achieve our desires, not just by attending church on Sundays. As Pfeifer points out towards the end of his book, for a Christian, healing should not be sought at *any* price. We should rather seek the will of God at any price. He asks rhetorically: "What is our primary focus? To be healed, or to glorify God in our life, no matter what He allows to happen to your body?"[1]

When modern medicine fails to meet our expectations, and treats us like machines, or when the bills exceed our budget, we may be tempted to try out alternative medicine. Its healers are kind, have plenty of time for each patient, are interested in our state of mind, not only in particular physical pain, fees are lower, the treatments are said to consist of natural, non-toxic ingredients, and last but not least, alternative medicine often

---

1. Pfeifer, *Healing at Any Price?*, 178.

Introduction

heals. If there were no real cases of healing, alternative medicine would discredit itself and disappear. There would be some naive or desperate people who would give it a try, but without results it could not survive. Perhaps you have already heard a success story, in terms of diagnosis or treatment, of a form of alternative medicine. Real cases of healing cannot be denied, and the placebo effect cannot be a sufficient explanation.[2]

After learning about how Eastern religions view the human person and having personally experienced several forms of alternative medicine, I noticed that its effectiveness had more to do with the spirituality of the Far East and New Age thinking than with medicine. So I decided to write this book from a Christian perspective with a special focus on understanding the spiritual grounds on which alternative medicine works. My intended readers are first of all Christians who are not sure what to make of the claims of alternative medicine. The second group I address are those who claim to be non-religious, but need to know that they embrace many quite religious beliefs by resorting to alternative medicine. And third, I am addressing healthcare professionals who want to understand the hidden mechanisms at work in alternative medicine. As far as I know, this topic is hardly mentioned in medical schools, and given the spread of these forms of "medicine," today's physicians need to know what "competition" offers.

Concerning the limitations of my approach, I must mention especially the following two: First, I do not refer to forms of alternative medicine that are not linked to spiritual beliefs, such as phytotherapy. Their effectiveness must be established through evidence-based medical research. If they do not poison us, their only potential danger is to postpone or reject a classic treatment, allowing an illness to worsen. This is a danger posed by any form of alternative medicine, regardless of its spiritual content. Second, I do not engage in the controversy of finding scientific proofs for the effectiveness or ineffectiveness of alternative medicine.[3] Again, this has to be established by medical research. My aim is of a different nature, that of investigating the spiritual dimension of alternative medicine, especially for the benefit of those who wish to be faithful Christians.

---

2. A placebo is a fake medication, with no real therapeutic effect (such as a sugar pill), which is given to a patient for its psychological benefit. It is commonly used in research to establish the value of a real drug, by comparing its effectiveness to such a placebo. The beneficial effect noticed when taking a placebo of a psychological origin, is called the placebo effect.

3. For a great resource on the medical effectiveness of alternative medicine see: O'Mathuna and Larimore, *Alternative Medicine*.

Introduction

A thorny issue for my inquiry concerns the position from which I analyze the spiritual dimension of alternative medicine. Which form of Christianity do I take as the standpoint? Rather than choose a single one, in the first chapter I seek to present a Christian position on human nature acceptable for both Catholics and Protestants, while Eastern Orthodox Christians should not feel excluded either. After all, there are more beliefs that unite us than those that divide us. Despite differences, we can find enough common theological ground in order to share a similar stand on alternative medicine.

The Bible[4] alone does not present us with a systematic treatise on human nature, so I turn to two other resources. For Catholics the reference point for formulating a position on human nature will obviously be the *Catechism of the Catholic Church*.[5] For Protestants I refer to the writings of the great Protestant theologian Karl Barth. When a certain doctrine is not common to both Catholics and Protestants, and a particular topic needs it, as for instance when assessing the idea of healing the soul through homeopathy, I will explain and use that doctrine. My aim is for all Christians to benefit from this book.

In the main part of the book (chapters 2 to 8), in light of the Christian teaching on human nature, I examine the views on human nature, health, and healing as they are defined in several of the best known forms of alternative medicine: Yoga, Ayurveda, anthroposophical medicine, acupuncture, reflexology, iridology, Reiki, therapeutic touch, macrobiotics, homeopathy, and Bach floral remedies. Finally, we reach conclusions and, it is hoped, acquire the skills for assessing the compatibility of any other form of alternative medicine with Christianity.

As you will learn in this book, alternative medicine is not just about healing. The stakes are much higher, as it leads one to ponder what is truly being healed, what mechanisms rule human nature, whether there is anything more to it than the illness of a physical body, and if so, what is the ultimate meaning of life. Such are the issues that concern the *spiritual* dimension of alternative medicine, which we should learn to discern.

Ernest Valea
December 9, 2019

    4. Bible quotations are from the *New Revised Standard Version* (NRSV).
    5. USCCB, *The Catechism of the Catholic Church* for the United States of America (abbreviated CCC), 1994. Only the numbers of the articles are mentioned in quotations.

1

Human Nature According to Christian Teaching

EVERY CHRISTIAN WOULD PROBABLY agree with the following article of the Catholic Catechism on human nature:

> The human person, created in the image of God, is a being at once corporeal and spiritual. The biblical account expresses this reality in symbolic language when it affirms that "then the LORD God formed man of dust from the ground, and breathed into his nostrils the breath of life; and man became a living being" (Genesis 2,7). Man, whole and entire, is therefore *willed* by God.[1]

There are two common philosophical views on human nature which are both wrong: physicalism, according to which we have a 100 percent material nature, and dualism (Cartesian, Platonic or Eastern), which asserts that the soul and the body are two fundamentally different substances. The right Christian view is that we are composed of one substance with two components: body and soul. They do not oppose each other (as in dualism); neither does the body exclude a spiritual component called the soul (as in physicalism). Barth emphasizes this important aspect of our nature, by stating:

> In sum, if materialism with its denial of the soul makes man subjectless, spiritualism with its denial of the body makes him objectless. Thus both result in a new and fatal division of man, although both are monistic in intention and the declared purpose of both

---

1. CCC 362.

is to demonstrate the unity of the human reality. But this demonstration may not be pursued at the cost of the reality of either of the two elements, reality being found either in body or soul and appearance either in soul or body.[2]

Given the intended readers of this book, I will not discuss reasons for rejecting the physicalist view, as all forms of alternative medicine deny that we have a strictly physical nature. However, it is vitally important to understand the shortcomings of the dualistic view, which considers the soul as a special substance that is temporarily located in a human body, uses it to achieve its goals and then abandons it at death.

According to Plato's philosophy, one of the oldest forms of dualism, the soul is a prisoner in the body, is reincarnated in many bodies according to its deeds in former lives, and must free itself from this bondage with the help of philosophy.[3] We find a similar idea in the many forms of Hinduism. If this is the relationship between the soul and the body, our life is a chance for the soul to escape its prison. But the Christian view of the human being is not dualistic. We are made of a single substance, with both a material and a spiritual component. In order to emphasize it, Barth rhetorically asks:

> If this is the case, if soul and body are two "parts" of which man is "composed," if these two "parts" are two self-contained substances, if these substances are quite different and even opposed in nature, and if this involves an opposition of the worth of the one (the soul) to the unworthiness of the other (the body), what are we to make of their alleged connexion and unity, and therefore of the unity of man's being ? (. . .) Is it not clear that in these circumstances soul and body neither have nor can have anything in common, but can only be in conflict and finally part from one another ?[4]

The Catholic Catechism also emphasizes that human nature consists of a single substance:

> The unity of soul and body is so profound that one has to consider the soul to be the 'form' of the body: i.e., it is because of its spiritual soul that the body made of matter becomes a living, human body; spirit and matter, in man, are not two natures united, but rather their union forms a single nature.[5]

---

2. Barth, *Church Dogmatics*, III,2, 392.
3. See Plato, *Phaedo* 82a-e, 285–89.
4. Barth, *Church Dogmatics*, III,2, 380.
5. CCC 365.

As a result, we need a way of understanding the relationship between body and soul that avoids both physicalism and dualism. I found it formulated by one of the greatest theologians of all time, Thomas Aquinas (1225–1274). Although he expressed his view on human nature as an adaptation of the philosophy of Aristotle, called hylomorphism,[6] he did not hellenize Christian thought. Rather, he Christianized Greek philosophy by using Aristotle's categories to teach Christian doctrine. In other words, although Aquinas used Aristotle's language to explain Christian teaching on human nature, he did not transform Christian theology into Greek philosophy, but expressed the truths of theology in the most appropriate philosophical language of his time.[7] This way of expressing Christian doctrine by the use of Greek categories should not bother Christians of any particular tradition, since the doctrine of the Holy Trinity itself was formulated by the use of neo-Platonic categories of *ousia* and *hypostasis* in the fourth century AD.

In order to grasp Aquinas's vision of human nature as a union of soul and body, we must first understand the two basic philosophical concepts he uses, those of form and matter. Any existing thing, whether living or non-living, is made up of matter and form. If we start from non-living things and take for example a stone, its matter consists of one or more minerals. In the case of a limestone rock, the raw matter is calcium carbonate—$CaCO_3$ (along with a number of impurities). The chemical substance called calcium carbonate can exist only under certain forms: as a piece of limestone, marble, chalk, or calcite. They all share $CaCO_3$ as raw material. Form is the concrete, individual way in which matter exists, and matter can only exist as configured by form.

In understanding living beings, we consider matter and form to be their body and soul. Plants and animals have bodies made up of many organic and inorganic substances, and the element that organizes these substances in the form of a tulip, a cat or a dog is the soul of that living being. The soul of a plant differs from that of an animal in that it possesses only the potential to feed itself, to grow, and to multiply, while the animal soul has the ability to feel and move. For this reason we say that the soul of a plant is vegetative, while that of the animal is sensitive.

The soul gives not only size, but also its essence, to matter. The soul is the element that makes it a member of a species. For example, if we analyze

---

6. The term comes from Greek, where *hyle* is *matter* and *morphē* is *form*.

7. We find his view on human nature thoroughly expounded in his *Summa Theologiae*, I, questions 75 to 102.

the differences between a cat and a dog from the point of view of the organic and inorganic substances out of which they are composed, they are almost identical. The same amino acids, fats, sugars, water, minerals, etc., are found in the constitution of both animals. The element that arranges them as a cat or a dog is the soul of that animal. A rough approximation of what the soul would be, in scientific terms, seems to be the DNA of that animal, for it dictates the formation of a specific organism out of basic organic and inorganic elements. But in Aquinas's view, the soul is more than that. A dead animal no longer has the potential to fulfill the functions of the living animal, because it no longer has that organizing principle called soul, although DNA is still there in every cell. According to Aquinas's vision, the corpse has another potential (another form), one that gives it the potential to break down into simple molecules. In other words, at death the soul is replaced by another form, with another potential. Once the plant or the animal dies, it ceases to exist as a living organism, which we express by saying that its soul does not survive death.

The human soul is different. If our soul were mortal like that of animals, we would follow the physicalist view of human nature. In order to grasp the right understanding of the Christian view of the human soul we need to place it in the context of a hierarchy in God's creation: nonliving matter, plants, animals, human beings, and angels. In the hierarchy of creation human beings are located between animals and angels. The highest category of creation are the angels, the immaterial beings defined as pure forms which do not configure matter. They are "purely spiritual," "personal and immortal," endowed with "intelligence and will."[8] From a physicalist point of view it is obvious that the existence of such beings cannot be accepted. But on physicalist premises neither can the existence of God be accepted. And since God exists as an immaterial supreme Being, both angels and human immaterial souls find their reason for being as God's special creation.

In the hierarchy of creation the nature of human beings resembles partly that of animals and partly that of angels. The animal soul configures the body but does not survive death, whereas angels are configured by God but do not configure a body. We resemble animals by having a material body configured by the soul, but also angels, by having a subsistent and immortal soul. In other words, we could say that humans have an amphibian nature; that is, we are living on the interface of the two worlds, and

---

8. CCC 330.

we participate in both. According to Christian teaching, the human soul is created by God at conception, configures the body, and survives death. Therefore, we are neither angels fallen into material bodies, in order to be purified of sins done in a pure spiritual world, according to Gnosticism, nor mammals that have evolved so much that they acquired self-consciousness, according to atheistic physicalism.

Although we affirm that the soul survives death, the Christian view of human nature is not a form of dualism, similar to Platonist or Hindu views. We are made of a single substance which consists of both body and soul. Although the soul survives its separation from the body, the state of the soul between death and resurrection does not define a complete human nature, for death was not God's plan for us. Death is the result of sin (according to Genesis 2:17). It is the separation of the soul from the body, and the state of the soul between death and resurrection is temporary. It is only at the resurrection that the soul becomes again part of a complete human substance. That is why we affirm in the Creed the resurrection of the body.

Another important aspect of the Christian view is that intellect and will are not simply powers of the brain (and therefore of the body), but of the immaterial soul. No matter how much progress we may see in the neurosciences, it is unthinkable that we will be able to understand the processes of the soul, that is, our most intimate thoughts, feelings, memories, and desires, as products of electrical fluxes between the billions of neurons in our cerebral cortex. In other words, it is unthinkable that we will ever be able to translate the electric impulses between neurons, of measurable electric intensity and frequency, into mind events such as memories, worries or holiday plans. The brain is undoubtedly linked to mental activity, being configured by the soul for that purpose, but it cannot be the true source of consciousness and personhood. The processes of the mind are of a different nature than those of the brain; they belong to the soul, which is of an immaterial and immortal nature.[9]

Given that dualism defines soul and body as different substances, the way the two substances interact, that is, how matter can inform the soul, or how the soul can influence matter, is very problematic. As we will see, this

---

9. The physicalist refusal to accept the soul as having a different nature from the body (and the brain) is a case of begging the question. The physicalist assumes that nothing immaterial can exist (neither God, nor angels); therefore neither can the immaterial soul. On this premise physicalism builds a view of human nature on 100 percent materialist terms, and then this philosophy is presented as an argument against the existence of the immaterial soul.

difficulty also arises in the spirituality proposed by some forms of alternative medicine, which is why they require an intermediate body, called the etheric body. But between two fundamentally different substances, a third one cannot serve as a bridge over the substantial gap. Dualism needs infinite intermediate bodies to bring a logical solution to how soul and body could interact. Aquinas was aware of this problem, encountered by the Platonists of his time, who also required the existence of an intermediary body. He says:

> If we suppose that the intellectual soul is not united to the body as its form, but only as its motor, as the Platonists maintain, it would necessarily follow that in man there is another substantial form, by which the body is established in its being as movable by the soul. If, however, the intellectual soul be united to the body as its substantial form, as we have said above (article 1), it is impossible for another substantial form besides the intellectual soul to be found in man.[10]

In conclusion, there are three important aspects we must remember in order to have the right picture on human nature: 1. We are not souls that use a body, but a unity of soul and body. 2. The soul is not a spiritual substance that can change bodies like clothes, as in Hinduism, for the union of the soul with the body is not accidental, but essential. 3. The body is not just a companion, instrument or container, from which the soul seeks to be released, but an essential component of human nature.

Another fundamental Christian doctrine we must be aware of is that God is not an impersonal force, or energy, that manifests human nature out of his essence, but a person who wishes to be in communion with us. In the words of Barth,

> The God of the Bible wills to be perceived, desired and loved in His visible, audible, tangible witnesses. (. . .) That is why He is described as the Other who can be perceived, desired and known by man (himself only a creature and not the Creator) in the midst of the created world.[11]

From the fact that God is a person who created us as persons, follows another important aspect that we need to understand of our nature, the fact that our soul does not have a divine nature. The soul is created by God out of nothing (*ex nihilo*), at conception. It does not "emanate" from

---

10. *Summa Theologiae*, I,76, art.7. The possibility that an intermediary would exist between the body and the soul is the topic of the ninth question of Aquinas's *Questions on the Soul*.

11. Barth, *Church Dogmatics*, III,2, 413.

God's nature, nor does the soul substantially "unite" with God after death. To quote Barth again,

> God does not in any sense belong to the constitution of man. God is neither a part nor the whole of human nature. He is identical neither with one of the elements of which in unity and order we are composed, nor with us ourselves."[12]

There is nothing in our nature that makes us immortal by itself. Our existence, as that of the material universe and of every other being, is sustained by God's grace. This is the natural consequence of the Christian concept of creation out of nothing. Barth emphasizes this aspect very clearly:

> Everything outside God is held constant by God over nothingness. Creaturely nature means existence in time and space, existence with a beginning and end, existence that becomes, in order to pass away again. Once it was and once it will no longer be.(. . .) The creature is threatened by the possibility of nothingness and of destruction, which is excluded by God—and only by God. If a creature exists, it is only maintained in its mode of existence if God so wills. If He did not so will, nothingness would inevitably break in from all sides. The creature itself could not rescue and preserve itself.[13]

Therefore we cannot speak of a "divine spark" or "a kernel of divinity" in our nature. This is a fundamental tenet that we must remember when analyzing the spiritual grounds of alternative medicine. We are created by God and totally dependent on him for our subsistence. Everything in God's creation, from atoms to angels, is being held in existence by God's grace. This is the correct framework for understanding human nature, and this understanding will keep us from heretical concepts of a "divine spark" that we allegedly have within us.

Once the Christian view of human nature has been clarified, we can start assessing the doctrines that lie at the core of various forms of alternative medicine and to what extent they can be reconciled with Christian teaching. Let us be guided by what both Catholic and Protestant theology teach on human nature. In Catholic terms we need to remember that:

> Being in the image of God the human individual possesses the dignity of a person, who is not just something, but someone. He

---

12. Barth, *Church Dogmatics*, III,2, 345.
13. Barth, *Dogmatics in Outline*, 55–56.

is capable of self-knowledge, of self-possession and of freely giving himself and entering into communion with other persons. And he is called by grace to a covenant with his Creator, to offer him a response of faith and love that no other creature can give in his stead.[14]

In a similar way, Barth says from a Protestant perspective:

> Just as man is distinguished from the rest of the created world by the fact that, as the likeness and promise of the divine covenant of grace, he is called to responsibility before God, so his special constitution corresponding to this calling is determined by the fact that he owes it to the God who is the Lord of this covenant of grace. This God as such is also the Creator of man. This God as such gives him his creatureliness. This God as such establishes him as soul and body, constituting the unity and order of this being, and maintaining him in this being in its unity and order.[15]

The question to bear in mind when dealing with a particular form of alternative medicine should thus be: Does its philosophical ground allow me to offer God a "response of faith and love," in a "covenant of grace," or does it rather lead me into a heretical view of God and human nature?

---

14. CCC 357.
15. Barth, *Church Dogmatics*, III,2, 347.

2

Yoga as Therapy and Religion

YOU HAVE PROBABLY HEARD of Yoga as a method of improving the quality of life by bringing both physical and psychological benefits ranging from weight loss to inner peace, and from joint flexibility to relief from stress and anxiety. Although its origin is found in Hinduism, its modern exponents present it as an ancient wisdom that goes beyond organized religion, or as an empirically developed science based on physiological mechanisms different from those of modern medicine. But if we carefully examine the tenets of Hinduism we will see that modern Yoga has a thoroughly religious ground, as it follows closely the ancient Hindu view of human nature.

Our aim in this chapter is to understand the nature of the self in Hinduism, the doctrine of reincarnation, the goal of Yoga practice, and the meaning of important Hindu notions such as the life-energy (*prana*), *kundalini*, and the *chakras*. This inquiry will provide the foundation for understanding the true nature of Yoga and the ground on which several forms of alternative medicine work. It will also help us assess to what extent this spiritual ground is compatible with Christianity.

2.1 ILLUSION, IGNORANCE, KARMA, AND REINCARNATION

Hinduism is not a single uniform religion, but rather a complex mixture of religious sects and philosophical schools in which we find pantheistic, dualistic, and theistic views, often difficult to systematize. In this chapter I will refer to pantheistic Hinduism, its most common form. Its origins can be traced in the Upanishads, a group of philosophical writings which appeared in the eighth and seventh centuries BC.[1] They teach that the world emerged as the manifestation of an impersonal essence called Brahman. In one of the earliest Upanishads we read:

> As a spider moves along the thread, as small sparks come forth from the fire, even so from this Self [Brahman] come forth all breaths, all worlds, all divinities, all beings.[2]

Unlike in the Christian representation of creation, which states that God created the world out of nothing (*ex nihilo*), in Hinduism the world is the transformation of an essence from one state (the unmanifested Brahman) into another state, which sums up all beings and non-living matter (the manifested Brahman). This is the philosophical ground of pantheism, the view that all particular beings in our world share in the essence of the ultimate reality. Human beings are one of the manifestations of this impersonal essence, along with gods, animals, plants, and matter. Like other living beings, we preserve in our nature a divine spark, an unaltered core which preserves Brahman's essence, and this core is the self (*atman*). It is not an equivalent of the Christian view of the soul, but is rather an impersonal entity that is changeless, inexpressible, eternal, and pure. The *Brihadaranyaka-Upanishad* states:

> The Self (*atman*) is not this, not this (*neti, neti*). He is incomprehensible, for he is not comprehended. He is indestructible, for he cannot be destroyed. He is unattached, for he does not attach himself. He is unfettered, he does not suffer, he is not injured.[3]

All beings are manifested from the impersonal Brahman and are meant to return to it, following a cycle that has no beginning and no end. A personal mode of existence has no ultimate fulfillment, for it is nothing but a wave on the ocean of being. Therefore, for Hindu pantheism the Christian view of everlasting life is absurd, a deception which keeps us from seeing how things really are.

---

1. Radhakrishnan, *The Principal Upanishads*, 22; Eliade, *A History of Religious Ideas*, I, 241.

2. *Brihadaranyaka-Upanishad* II,1,20, in Radhakrishnan, *The Principal Upanishads*, 190.

3. *Brihadaranyaka-Upanishad* IV,2,4, in Radhakrishnan, *The Principal Upanishads*, 254.

Illusion (*maya*) is the great deceiver about our true nature, as it channels our attention and desires towards the phenomenal world. Illusion generates ignorance (*avidya*), the inability to know the truth of how things really are, and ignorance triggers a spiritual law called karma, a law of cause and effect in the spiritual world that forces the self to bear the consequences of ignorance in one's present life and in future lives. This is, in short, the justification for reincarnation (*samsara*), which is the practical way in which one collects the fruits of his or her deeds in a new existence as a human being, a god, a ghost or an animal. As a result of karma, any human action has a precise and inevitable effect on its doer. The Indian philosopher T.M.P. Mahadevan explains:

> The group into which a soul is born is determined by the soul's past karma. The soul is born as an animal if there is an excess of demerit, as a god if there is an excess of merit, and as a human being if there is a balance between merit and demerit.[4]

The first clear affirmation of reincarnation is found in the *Brihadaranyaka-Upanishad*, which states that "one becomes good by good action, bad by bad action."[5] What one becomes, that is, the future life and the sorrows and joys that accompany it, is the result of the desires we follow in our ignorance. As we can read in the same Upanishad, "a person consists of desires. As is his desire so is his will; as is his will, so is the deed he does, whatever deed he does, that he attains."[6] The "desire" that generates one's becoming is that of experiencing the physical world and, consequently, illusion, and "the deed he does" is the seed of ignorance sown in this life, which will bear fruit in a future life. However, the "deeds" and "desires" that fuel karma are not just the bad ones, like those which Christians call sins. Karma and reincarnation is not just a means of "punishing" evil deeds and desires. Karma is an impersonal law, which also "rewards" good deeds and as such *all* deeds prolong the vicious cycle illusion—ignorance—karma—reincarnation. The *Mundaka Upanishad* affirms:

> Since those who perform rituals do not understand (the truth) because of attachment, therefore they sink down, wretched, when

---

4. Mahadevan, *Invitation to Indian Philosophy*, 391.

5. *Brihadaranyaka-Upanishad* III, 2,13, in Radhakrishnan, *The Principal Upanishads*, 217. Mircea Eliade argues that the term *samsara* does not appear in texts earlier than the Upanishads (Eliade, *A History of Religious Ideas*, I, 239).

6. *Brihadaranyaka-Upanishad* IV,4,5, in Radhakrishnan, *The Principal Upanishads*, 272.

their worlds (that is, the fruits of their merits) are exhausted. These deluded men, regarding sacrifices and works of merits as most important, do not know any other good. Having enjoyed in the high place of heaven won by good deeds, they enter again this world or a still lower one.[7]

2.2 HUMAN NATURE AND LIBERATION

In the *Taittiriya Upanishad* we find the oldest account of human nature as a construct of five layers (or sheaths): the physical (*annamaya*), formed by food; the vital (*pranamaya*), formed by breath; the mind (*manomaya*); the intellect (*vijnanamaya*); and finally the sheath of bliss (*anandamaya*), in which the self (*atman*) rests.[8] The physical layer is what we see, touch and heal by recourse to Western medicine, while the others are not the subject of scientific inquiry. According to Hindu philosophy and many forms of alternative medicine, the physical body is kept alive by an unseen body made of vital energy. This is the *pranamaya kosha*. It taps the universal life-energy called *prana*, and distributes it to the physical body. As the Indian master Vivekananda points out, *prana* represents the energy which sustains all physical and mental processes:

> Out of this *Prana* is evolved everything that we call energy, everything that we call force. It is the *Prana* that is manifesting as motion; it is the *Prana* that is manifesting as gravitation, as magnetism. It is the *Prana* that is manifesting as the actions of the body, as the nerve currents, as thought force. From thought down to the lowest force, everything is but the manifestation of *Prana*. The sum total of all forces in the universe, mental or physical, when resolved back to their original state, is called *Prana*.[9]

The next two layers are mental. *Manomaya* is formed by perception, the result of sense activity, while *vijnanamaya* is formed by reasoning and interpreting in a subjective way the data of perception. Finally, *anandamaya* is the layer that serves as a bridge between the other-worldly self (*atman*) and the other four layers.

---

7. Mundaka Upanishad I, 2,9–10, in Radhakrishnan, *The Principal Upanishads*, 677.

8. Taittiriya Upanishad II.1, in Radhakrishnan, *The Principal Upanishads*, 541–43.

9. Vivekananda, *Lectures on Raja Yoga*, 31. Swami Vivekananda was one of the first Hindu missionaries to the United States. He gave lectures on Yoga at the World's Columbian Exposition in Chicago in 1893.

In Vedanta, the pantheistic philosophy which emerged from the Upanishads, these five layers form three bodies: the gross body (*sthula sarira*), made of the physical layer; the subtle body (*sukshma sarira*), made of the next three; and the causal body (*karana sarira*), the one that holds the self. This last body is the location where karmic imprints are stored, as this body, unlike the other two, follows the self to its next incarnation. The karmic imprints in the causal body will materialize unconsciously in a future life, without giving any clue for understanding what we owe to past lives. By no means can it be a conscious memory.

The self can attain liberation only while experiencing a human existence, which is why we enjoy a privileged position in the hierarchy of beings. Our position is more privileged even than that of the gods, for they represent the stage of harvesting positive merits of a human existence, while animals represent the other extreme, that of harvesting the fruit of negative merit. One should not miss the opportunity to stop the cycle of reincarnation, and make every effort to end the perpetuation of ignorance and attain liberation. The ultimate possible accomplishment of human existence is thus releasing the self from reincarnation and its merging with Brahman, like a droplet of water that falls into the ocean and becomes one with it. The *Mundaka Upanishad* uses a similar image:

> Just as the flowing rivers disappear in the ocean casting off name
> and shape, even so the knower, freed from name and shape, attains
> to the divine person, higher than the high.[10]

Pantheism has no place for personal fulfillment of human nature in this life or in an everlasting life, as in the Christian view of heaven. Personal existence is synonymous with suffering, and therefore the way out of suffering is the abolition of our personal nature.

2.3 HOW MUCH RELIGION IS IN YOGA?

In order to achieve liberation, one must follow an ascetic and meditative path that breaks the bondage of ignorance and karma. The general term used for designating such an ascetic path is Yoga.[11] In the present technical sense, the term "Yoga" is first used in the *Taittiriya* and *Katha Upanishads*

---

10. Mundaka Upanishad III,2,8–9, in Radhakrishnan, *The Principal Upanishads*, 691.

11. According to Eliade, "The word *yoga* serves, in general, to designate any *ascetic technique* and any *method of meditation*" (Eliade, *Yoga: Immortality and Freedom*, 4).

(around the fifth century BC). In the latter, the god of death (Yama) teaches the young Naciketas how to acquire the knowledge of Brahman through restraint of the senses and concentration.[12] Using an interesting allegory, he likens the human body to a chariot pulled by wild horses (the senses) that the driver (the mind) cannot master. In this chariot, the passenger (the self) suffers in silence. Yoga is the method by which the driver (the mind) can calm and stop the horses (the senses) so that the passenger (*atman*) can descend from the chariot.

The most widespread Yoga school today is Hatha Yoga. It is promoted in the West as an effective relaxation method and health therapy. Most Westerners are aware only of its physical aspect, the body postures, which would suggest it is a kind of gymnastics for health. However, its postures, twists and bends are only preparatory stages for enabling meditation. In the very first verse of the *Hatha Yoga Pradipika* of Svatmarama,[13] the fundamental treatise of *Hatha Yoga*, this goal is very clearly affirmed: "Reverence to Shiva the Lord of Yoga, who taught [his wife] Parvati *hatha* wisdom as the first step to the pinnacle of *raja yoga*." *Raja yoga* means here the practice of meditation, meant to liberate the mind from illusion and achieve final liberation:

> When the mind becomes unified, this is *raja yoga*. The yogi, now master of creation and destruction, becomes one with God. Whether or not you call it liberation, here is eternal bliss. The bliss of dissolution [*laya*] is obtained only through *raja yoga*. There are many who are merely hatha yogis, without the knowledge of raja yoga. They are simple practitioners who will never reap the [real] fruits of their efforts.[14]

B.K.S. Iyengar, the well-known Yoga teacher in the West, points out that Yoga is much more than a relaxation method. In his words, it is "the union of the individual self, *jivatma*, with the universal self, *paramatma*."[15] As he further explains, the word *yoga* itself points to its religious content:

> The word "Yoga" is derived from the Sanskrit root "*yuj*" which means to bind, join, attach and yoke, to direct and concentrate

---

12. *Katha Upanishad* I,3,3–9, in Radhakrishnan, *The Principal Upanishads*, 623–24.

13. B.K.S. Iyengar, a well known Yoga teacher, argues it was composed as late as the fifteenth century AD (Iyengar, *Yoga*, 48), about the same time as the *Gheranda Samhita* (Iyengar, *Yoga*, 53).

14. Svatmarama, *The Hathayogapradipika* IV,77.

15. Iyengar, *Yoga*, 46.

the attention in order to use it for meditation. (...) It is the communion of the human soul with Divinity.[16]

Therefore Yoga cannot be reduced to a method of coping with daily stress. Iyengar makes it very clear that Yoga "systematically teaches man to search for the divinity within himself with thoroughness and efficiency. He unravels himself from the external body to the self within,"[17] thus leading not only to flexibility and inner peace, but also "from death to immortality."[18]

The underlying philosophy attached to Hatha Yoga practice is a form of pantheistic Hinduism. Brahman and *atman* are presented under different names, but bear the same meaning as in the Upanishads. The ultimate reality is the god Shiva who, together with his divine consort, the goddess Shakti, form a state of primordial unity that corresponds to the Brahman of the Upanishads.[19] The world and the human beings appeared by the undoing of that primordial unity between Shiva and Shakti. The *Shiva-Samhita* states:

> From the self-combination of the Spirit which is Shiva and the Matter which is Shakti, and, through their inherent interaction on each other, all creatures are born.[20]

As the Upanishads assert that Brahman's pure essence is found in us as *atman*, similarly in Hatha Yoga (and in Tantra), we are said to have a divine core called the *kundalini*. It represents Shakti dissociated from her original unity with Shiva, and thus the ultimate goal of Hatha Yoga practice is the restoration of their unity for each individual human being. Hatha Yoga is thus a way of achieving the return of the self (Shakti, corresponding to *atman*) in the Absolute Shiva (corresponding to Brahman).[21] This means the abolition of personal existence, the same goal stated by the Upanishads and all forms of pantheism. In the words of Iyengar,

> The experience of *samadhi* [liberation] is achieved when the knower, the knowable, and the known become one. When the

---

16. Iyengar, *Light on Pranayama*, 4.
17. Iyengar, *Light on Pranayama*, 5.
18. Iyengar, *Light on Pranayama*, 5.
19. The word *hatha* is composed of two syllables: *ha*—sun, and *tha*—moon. Hatha designates the need to unite these two principles, which correspond to Shiva and Shakti.
20. *Shiva-Samhita* I,92.
21. In left-handed Tantra the reunion of the two principles is attained by unorthodox practices which include the sexual union of a man who embodies Shiva, and a woman, who embodies Shakti.

object of meditation engulfs the meditator and becomes the subject, self-awareness is lost.[22]

2.4 HATHA YOGA PRACTICE AND ITS DEFINING ELEMENTS

According to Timothy McCall, one of Iyengar's disciples, the practice of Yoga can

> reduce stress, increase flexibility, improve balance, promote strength, heighten cardiovascular conditioning, lower blood pressure, reduce overweight, strengthen bones, prevent injuries, lift mood, improve immune function, increase the oxygen supply to the tissues, heighten sexual functioning and fulfillment, foster psychological equanimity, and promote spiritual well-being . . . and that's only a partial list.[23]

Timothy McCall is one of many Yoga teachers who present Yoga as devoid of religion and fit for any practitioner, religious or not. He says: "Yoga is not a religion. Although yoga came out of ancient India it is not a form of Hinduism. In fact, yoga is happily practiced by Christians, Buddhists, Jews, Muslims, atheists, and agnostics alike."[24] He is partially right here, as Yoga is indeed practiced by Christians and adherents of other religions. But the other part is misleading, for Yoga came out of India as applied Hinduism. McCall admits that "there is certainly a spiritual side to yoga" but argues that one has the option to not "subscribe to any particular beliefs to benefit from it."[25] However, it is easy to see that Yoga devoid of its religious content is no longer Yoga.

The practice of physical postures (the *asanas*) is not just a form of Indian gymnastics for gaining physical health, vigor, mental balance, etc., but a way of gaining control over the body in order to enable the practice of meditation, and finally, to achieve liberation. As such it has a much deeper function than seeking physical mobility, relaxation, or any of its other indicated health benefits.

The beneficial effects on bodily health are due to physical exercise, but *asana* has a much deeper meaning than simple physical exercise. Iyengar

---

22. Iyengar, *Yoga*, 53.
23. McCall, *Yoga as Medicine*, 3.
24. McCall, *Yoga as Medicine*, 7.
25. McCall, *Yoga as Medicine*, 7.

points out that the *asanas* "help to transform an individual by bringing him or her away from the awareness of the body toward the consciousness of the soul."[26] This does not, however, refer to the soul in the Christian sense, but to the *atman*, the Hindu view of the self. So to use Yoga just for health and relaxation is like using this book as a fly swatter. It will work for a while. But sooner or later you will destroy it, for it is not intended for that use. In a similar way, Yoga can bring physical and psychological benefits, but only as a secondary result, for its primary goal is liberation in the Hindu sense.

The other well-known part of Yoga practice is the control of breathing, *pranayama*. But here again, we are dealing with a spiritual view of breathing, not the mere enhancing of our breathing efficiency. Iyengar defines *prana* as "the energy permeating the universe at all levels," "prime mover of all activity," "energy which creates, protects and destroys," "the principle of life and consciousness," "the breath of all beings in the universe."[27] Therefore we can understand that the control of breathing in Yoga is meant to control the exchange of *prana* between the body and the environment.[28] As Iyengar argues, the body postures are an aid for this stage of Yoga practice: "The practice of *asanas* removes the obstructions which impede the flow of *prana*."[29] Since mental activity is also sustained by *prana*, its respiratory intake must be controlled as strictly as possible in order to bring the mind under control. This is the higher level of Yoga, the level of achieving oneness with ultimate reality.

As mentioned in the previous section, in Hatha Yoga and Tantra the self is the spiritual entity called *kundalini*. In the words of Iyengar, it is "the divine, cosmic energy which exists as a latent force in everyone."[30] The *kundalini* lies dormant at the base of the main spiritual channel (*nadi*)[31] that traverses the body. This channel is called *sushumna*. Its starting point corresponds to the base of the spine, and the end point is located at the top of the head. The whole ascetic practice aims at "awakening" the *kundalini* and its rise through the *sushumna nadi* from its base to its top. Parallel to

---

26. Iyengar, *Yoga*, 48.

27. Iyengar, *Light on Pranayama*, 12.

28. According to Iyengar, "*Prana* is energy, and *ayama* is the storing and distribution of that energy" (Iyengar, *Yoga*, 54).

29. Iyengar, *Yoga*, 54.

30. Iyengar, *Yoga*, 54.

31. The *nadis* are the channels through which *prana* circulates. The *Shiva Samhita* says there are 350,000 such channels (Iyengar, *Light on Pranayama*, 33).

the *sushumna*, on its left and right side, are the *ida* and *pingala nadis*. Their starting point is at the base of the spine and the upper end corresponds to the two nostrils. *Ida* and *pingala* are the main channels which transport *prana*. Therefore, in the Hatha Yoga technique of breath control (*pranayama*), at inspiration (*puraka*), the right nostril is closed with a finger and air is inspired through the left nostril (which corresponds to the *ida* channel), one holds his or her breath (*kumbhaka*), and then the left nostril is closed and air is expired (*rechaka*) through the right nostril which corresponds to the *pingala* channel.

According to Hatha Yoga practice, by the control of breathing and meditation one achieves the awakening and ascension of *kundalini* through the *sushumna* channel. On its way it meets seven important points, called *chakras*. They have a very important role, both in Yoga practice and in several forms of alternative medicine. According to Iyengar, "Just as the brain controls physical, mental, and intellectual functions through the nerve cells or neurons, *chakras* tap the *prana* or cosmic energy which is within all living beings and transform it into spiritual energy. This is spread through the body by the *nadis*, or channels."[32]

The *chakras* are located along the *sushumna* channel, as follows:

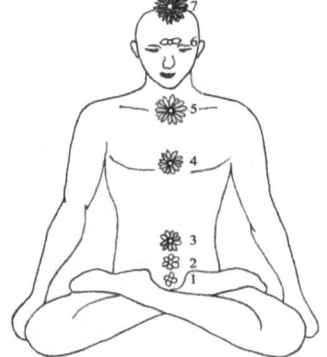

1. at the base of the spine is the *muladhara-chakra*. It is the place where *kundalini* lies dormant in all ignorant people;[33]

2. a short distance above the first is the *svadhishtana-chakra*;

3. near the navel is the *manipura-chakra*;

4. near the heart is the *anahata-chakra*;

5. at the base of the neck is the *vishuddha-chakra*;

6. between the eyebrows is the *ajna-chakra* (also called the "spiritual eye" or the "third eye");

7. at the top of the head and the end of the *sushumna* channel is the *sahasrara-chakra* (also called "the one-thousand petals lotus").

---

32. Iyengar, *Yoga*, 57.
33. It lies coiled as a snake and for this reason it also called the *kundalini* snake.

When the *kundalini* has traversed the entire *sushumna* channel and reaches the last *chakra* as a result of a successful Yoga practice, one experiences liberation, the ultimate goal of Yoga practice.

2.5 YOGA AND ITS ESOTERIC POWERS AND EXPERIENCES

A form of Yoga close to Hatha Yoga, which emphasizes the awakening and rising of the *kundalini*, is Siddha Yoga.[34] It stresses the importance of being led by a guru[35] and to rely on his or her power for spiritual awakening. Unlike in Hatha Yoga, in which the practitioner's effort is intense, and the guru only serves as a mentor, in Siddha Yoga, it is the master who triggers the awakening of *kundalini*. The *Hatha Yoga Pradipika* affirms of this option:

> When the *kundalini* is sleeping it will be aroused by the grace of the guru. Then all the *chakras* and knots are pierced and *prana* flows through the royal road of *sushumna*. The mind is released from its work and the yogi conquers death."[36]

The "grace" received from the guru is different from what Christians mean by grace. It is the power given by the guru either by revealing a secret mantra, by a touch on the forehead (the place of the *ajna chakra*), or even by a simple glance. The act of initiation itself, said to be a transfer of spiritual energy from master to disciple, is called *Shaktipat*. Disciples have experienced intense physical manifestations occurring at the awakening and rising of *kundalini* through the "grace" of the master. Ajit Mookerjee mentions the following experiences:

- creeping sensations in the spinal cord;
- tingling sensations all over the body;
- automatic and involuntary laughing or crying;
- hearing unusual noises;
- seeing visions of deities or saints;
- constriction of breathing, seeming sometimes to cease altogether;

---

34. It is also called Kundalini Yoga, Shakti Yoga or Shaktipat Yoga.
35. The guru is the master who leads his or her disciple from ignorance to enlightenment, or in other words, from darkness (*gu*) to light (*ru*).
36. *Hatha Yoga Pradipika*, III, 2–3.

- spontaneous chanting of mantras or songs, or simply vocal noises;
- performing *asanas* both known and unknown;
- shaking, trembling and becoming limp, or turning as rigid as stone.[37]

When such manifestations occur, disciples are reassured that they are normal signs that "*Kundalini* Shakti has become active."[38] Some of them are also experienced in Reiki, in which the most usual and expected is the flow of energy from the crown *chakra* through the whole body, to the palms. Along with such sensations disciples can experience so-called paranormal powers (*siddhis*), hence the name of this practice—Siddha Yoga.[39] The *Yoga Sutra* mentions the following paranormal powers (*siddhis*) which prove the spiritual progress of the practitioner: a deep comprehension of past and future events (III,16), knowledge of former births (III,18), the condition of other people's minds (III,19), the ability to become invisible (III,21), the knowledge of the moment of one's death (III,23), the acquisition of paranormal physical power (III,24–25), clairvoyance (III,26), entering into the body of another person (III,39), levitation (III,40), etc.[40]

In books on spiritual awakening, as well as in testimonies of practitioners, not infrequently the appearance of spiritual beings during meditation has been witnessed. For example, Swami Sivananda (1887–1963), one of the most important Hindu missionaries to the West, mentions both the appearance of benevolent spirits:

> You will see your Ishta Devata or tutelary deity in handsome dress with four hands and weapons. Siddhas (perfected masters), Rishis (Hindu sages) and other Devatas (gods) appear before you to encourage you. You will find a huge collection of Devatas and celestial ladies with various musical instruments in their hands.[41]

and that of evil spirits or fearful apparitions:

> Sometimes, these elementals appear during meditation. They are strange figures, some with long teeth, some with big faces, some with big bellies, some with faces on the belly and some with faces

---

37. Mookerjee, *Kundalini*, 71–72.
38. Mookerjee, *Kundalini*, 72.
39. The *Yoga Sutra* is an exposition of the *Yoga-darshana* of Patanjali, one of the six orthodox philosophical schools of Hinduism.
40. Patanjali, *Yoga Sutra*, 174–93.
41. Sivananda, *Practice of Yoga*, 226.

on the head. They are inhabitants of the *Bhuta Loka*. They are the attendants of Lord Shiva. They have terrifying forms.[42]

Far from being a worrying element, meeting such spirits is desirable, as they can further lead the Yoga practitioner to deeper spiritual achievement:

> The beings and objects with whom you are in touch during the early period of meditation belong to the astral world. They are similar to human beings minus a physical overcoat. (. . .) The lustrous forms are higher Devatas of mental or higher planes, who come down to give you Darshana and encourage you. Various Shaktis manifest themselves in lustrous forms. Adore them. Worship them.[43]

All the above paranormal powers and visualizations of spirits are said to be mere stages of one's spiritual evolution. One does not need to worry or be afraid, but to advance steadily to the ultimate goal, which is union with the ultimate reality, Brahman. As Sivananda affirms: "The highest goal or realization is profound Silence or Supreme Peace, wherein all thoughts cease and you become identical; with the Supreme Self."[44]

For a Christian, however, meeting such spirits should cause major concern. Since they encourage following a spiritual path that is adverse to Christian teaching (the loss of personal status through reunion with ultimate reality), they must be demons. The apostle Paul warns us that "Even Satan disguises himself as an angel of light. So it is not strange if his ministers also disguise themselves as ministers of righteousness" (2 Cor 11,14–15). Therefore we must be aware that a Christian can be deceived by such spirits, and following a spirit guide will eventually lead to the loss of faith.

2.6 CHAKRA HEALING

The *chakras* play an important role not only in Hatha Yoga, but also in many forms of alternative medicine. Ayurveda and Reiki are two of the best known. While in Yoga they are gates through which the *kundalini* rises on its way to liberation, in Hindu-related forms of alternative medicine they

---

42. Sivananda, *Concentration and Meditation*, 321. One should not be scared by such devilish apparitions. Sivananda reassures: "They do not cause any harm at all. They simply appear on the stage. They come to test your strength and courage" (Sivananda, *Concentration and Meditation*, 321).

43. Sivananda, *Practice of Yoga*, 227.

44. Sivananda, *Concentration and Meditation*, 354.

are said to control our health by assuring the flow of *prana* to the organs of our body. Therefore when one of the organs malfunctions, the corresponding *chakra* needs to be charged, or "balanced," in order to better capture and distribute spiritual energy. This "recharging" or "balancing" is done in several ways.

The first is of course Yoga, by its postures, breathing control and meditation. Another is Reiki therapy, which constitutes a separate chapter of this book. A third one is *chakra* meditation, a way of focusing on each *chakra* and balancing its energy flow by sending positive thoughts to it until the right flow is reestablished. A variant or aid to this technique is the use of mantras. While it is generally said that mantras produce the right "spiritual frequency" that adjusts the energy flow, we need to know that in Hinduism mantras have a deep spiritual meaning.[45]

A fourth method is color therapy. It is said to work on the assumption that each *chakra* is linked to a certain color of the rainbow (from the first to the seventh: red, orange, yellow, green, blue, indigo and violet). Exposing the body to light of one of these colors will balance the energy of the corresponding *chakra*. Although it appears to have some scientific aura, color therapy is nothing but Hindu spirituality under the guise of science. Since *chakras* belong to a "subtle body" known only in worldviews of Hindu origin, there is no link between *chakra* healing and medical science. By no means could we imagine how a physical phenomenon, such as light, can interfere or interact with a non-physical energy, such as *prana*, and with non-physical elements as the *chakras*.

The fifth of the associated spiritual therapies associated with *chakra* healing is crystal (or healing stones) therapy. Its working principle lies on the assumption that certain crystals (such as quartz, amethyst, fluorite, tourmaline, etc.) can tap spiritual energy directly from the external world and direct it towards the *chakra* upon which it has been laid. For instance, a quartz crystal laid over an imbalanced *anahata-chakra* can heal the heart of physical ailments such as angina (chest pain). Color healing and crystal healing can be associated, given that crystals have certain colors. The most important is said to be quartz, able to heal multiple *chakras*. Depending on the practitioner, one or more stones can be laid on each *chakra*. Although the use of crystals for healing looks like a nature-friendly therapy (the purity of nature at work for our health), its *modus operandi* is esoteric, linked directly to worldviews of Hindu origin.

45. I will return to this topic in chapter 4, on Ayurveda.

2.7 YOGA FOR CHRISTIANS?

Yoga and *chakra*-healing have in common the fact that they fuel a view of human nature that corresponds to Hindu spirituality. Contrary to Christian teaching, human life is no longer the gift of God, but a flow of cosmic energy that needs to be balanced in order to attain oneness with the universe. The belief that our soul is a spark of divinity is a flat denial of Christian teaching, as we were created out of nothing and are held in existence solely by the grace of God. Nothing and no one except God has a divine nature. The union of the soul with the essence of God (as the *atman*-Brahman view of liberation) is thus an impossible tenet for a Christian. We are meant to be everlasting persons in communion with God in an everlasting bond of love, in which we remain separate persons. In other words, Christian salvation is a perfection of love of the individual human person in communion with God, not an impersonal merging with him.

Could one ignore the esoteric ground of Yoga and practice it as an ancient form of Indian gymnastics, devoid of any "spiritual" content? Although many teachers claim to follow this non-religious view, Yoga can hardly work as gymnastics. First, a practice of Yoga without recourse to its defining elements such as the self, liberation, *prana*, *kundalini* and *chakras*, is meaningless. It is no longer Yoga. Second, it does not have the same "healing" effect for one who does not follow its real goal, that of achieving awakening and liberation. One may feel some physical improvement, but one cannot get too far in the ability to perform the more complicated *asanas* without breath control and meditation. The guru himself may indicate that in order to advance in the skill to perform *asanas* it is necessary to start meditation.

As with many other forms alternative medicine, once a person feels some improvement to health as a result of Yoga practice he or she may become curious to know the deeper grounds of this "gymnastics" and start believing the spirituality associated with it. Although the guru may say that it is possible for one to keep his or her Christian faith, one who starts meditation gradually embraces more and more of the esoteric beliefs of Hinduism, like the divine self, karma, and reincarnation. Once these are accepted, one becomes a follower of Hinduism and his or her "old-fashioned" Christian faith is lost. This is the true danger of Yoga practice. It is the loss of saving faith, of no longer being able to offer God "a response of faith and love" and become a responsible partner in "a covenant of grace."

2.8 REINCARNATION AND CHRISTIANITY

Since the belief in reincarnation is part of many forms of alternative medicine, we need to remind ourselves at this point of the main reasons why it cannot be reconciled to Christianity. In Hinduism reincarnation is the result of karma and ignorance, of not being able to achieve the impersonal fusion of the self with its source. To attain spiritual enlightenment means to break the bondage of ignorance by no longer clinging to the thirst of experiencing personal existence. As Eliade argues, "human personality does not exist as a final element; it is only a synthesis of psychomental experiences, and it is destroyed – in other words, ceases to act – as soon as revelation is an accomplished fact."[46]

The "modern" view of reincarnation differs substantially from the Hindu one. Far from being considered a torment, from which we must escape by all means, even at the cost of the abolition of our personal status, reincarnation has become an eternal progression of the soul to higher spiritual existences. This adaptation to modern Western thought was accomplished mainly by the Theosophical Society, founded by Helena Blavatsky (1831–1891), and by Anthroposophy, founded by Rudolf Steiner (1861–1925). As a result of their efforts, of the many Eastern gurus who have since visited and moved to the Western world, and of New Age spirituality, reincarnation has become one of the most popular explanations of the origin and meaning of life.

Under the influence of a Western religious context, dominated by monotheistic religions, but in contradiction to Hinduism, today we hear that what reincarnates is our soul, which keeps the attributes of personhood from one incarnation to the next. This compromise follows the need to adapt Eastern teachings to the expectations of Western people. We will see this expressed in the teachings of Rudolf Steiner, the founder of Anthroposophy and its associated form of medicine.

Further attempts to accommodate reincarnation to Western thought are made by asserting that reincarnation can be found in the Bible and in the writings of the Church Fathers; that it was forbidden only as late as at the Second Council of Constantinople (553 AD); and that it has been

---

46. Eliade, *Yoga*, 31. A few pages later he adds: "Once it is granted that this freedom cannot be gained in our present human condition and that personality is the vehicle of suffering and drama, it becomes clear that what must be sacrificed is the human condition and the 'personality.' And this sacrifice is lavishly compensated for by the conquest of absolute freedom, which it makes possible" (Eliade, *Yoga*, 35.).

proven by hypnotic regression as well as by stories of children who tell of their previous lives. I will not address these issues here, because a more comprehensive assessment of such "proofs" is needed, which goes beyond the scope of this book.[47] I will, however, reiterate the main reasons why Christians cannot accept reincarnation.

First, reincarnation undermines God's sovereignty over his creation, turning him into a powerless spectator to human suffering. The problem of suffering does not require karma and reincarnation as its solution. God can punish evil and will do it in a perfect way at the end of history.[48] Regardless of the difficulty of the situation in which a Christian finds himself or herself, God knows about it and allows it for a higher purpose. He allows evil for our ultimate good, according to each one's ability to cope with it.[49] Christianity does not need karma as a cosmic legislator, because this role belongs solely to the eternal God who created us and keeps us in existence.

Second, belief in reincarnation can jeopardize one's understanding of morality and motivation for moral living. One living consistently with belief in reincarnation should not be troubled by the occurrence of murder, rape, theft, and other such social plagues, since they should be seen as results of debts coming from the past lives of their victims. In the same way tragedies of past and present wars should be considered nothing more than a fulfillment of karmic justice. Any involvement in helping the "victims" of karma would only delay the application of its requirements. Therefore belief in reincarnation can undermine motivation for morality and virtue, encouraging passivity instead of involvement for the well-being of our neighbor.

Third, reincarnation contradicts the way human nature is defined in Christianity as a unity of soul and body. The human soul is created individually by God to animate a single *human* body. After death it cannot move into the body of an animal or another human being, for it awaits resurrection.

Fourth, reincarnation threatens the very essence of the Christian doctrine of salvation, which affirms the necessity of Jesus' sacrifice for our salvation. The apostle Peter boldly taught his disciples:

> He himself bore our sins in his body on the cross, so that, free from sins, we might live for righteousness; by his wounds you have been healed (1 Pet 2,24).

---

47. This is my next project, which I hope will follow soon.
48. See Matt 25,31–46, Rev 20,10–15.
49. See 1 Cor 10,13.

If we need to pay for our sins in future lives to gain salvation according to the requirements of karma, Jesus' crucifixion would be irrelevant and absurd. It would no longer be the only solution for our salvation, but only a terrible accident in human history. Moreover, we would have to believe that Jesus died on the cross as a punishment for his own sins committed in his previous lives. And as for what he did in those "former lives" to merit such a cruel death, it is impossible to imagine where speculation might lead. Therefore, no matter how much "evidence" could be brought to support reincarnation, it is doomed to fail in the attempt to be reconciled with Christianity.

Once we have understood how human nature is defined in both Christian and Hindu spirituality, we can now move on to analyzing two forms of alternative medicine with strong Hindu attachments: Ayurveda and anthroposophic medicine.

3

Anthroposophical Medicine (AM)

RUDOLF STEINER (1861–1925) IS the founder of the Anthroposophical Society (in short, anthroposophy), a Gnostic worldwide movement, whose views have been applied to many domains, ranging from philosophy and religion to pedagogy, architecture, art, social sciences, agriculture, and last but not least, medicine. Steiner's spiritual formation is very complex. He was heavily influenced by the esotericism promoted by Goethe, as well as by Schopenhauer and by Nietzsche's theory of the overman (*Übermensch*). The most important source of his spiritual formation, however, was the Theosophical Society, a movement founded in 1875 in the United States by Helena Blavatsky and Henry Olcott to promote the study of esoteric philosophies, Eastern religions, occultism, and the unity of religions. In 1902 Steiner became the General Secretary of the German branch of Theosophy and directed it towards the study of Western esoteric and Gnostic traditions. He came into conflict with the headquarters of Theosophy in Madras (India) when he opposed Krishnamurti's promotion as a great initiate that would inaugurate a new era in world spirituality. This caused Steiner to break from the parent organization in 1913 and found a new one, the Anthroposophical Society.

Steiner was a very prolific author. He wrote dozens of books and held hundreds of conferences throughout Europe. Anthroposophical medicine is the application of his ideas in medicine, a new domain in which his closest colleague and co-founder was Ita Wegman (1876–1943). This branch of alternative medicine is formulated on complicated esoteric theories of the relationship between human beings and the universe, the need for spiritual evolution and reincarnation, the relationship between four components of human nature, and the interaction between seven planets, seven metals, and their "correspondents" in internal organs.

3.1 THE FOUR COMPONENTS OF HUMAN NATURE

Ita Wegman argues that AM is not opposed "to modern (homogenic) medicine which is working with scientific methods."[1] The difference is that AM adds "a further knowledge, whose discoveries are made by different methods,"[2] coming from a world whose laws "are different, in fact, the very opposite to those of the physical world."[3] One of these "different" laws that modern medicine does not know is karma. It can bring bad health in this life from previous lives following a similar logic we have seen operating in Hinduism. In Steiner's words, for a true healing "we have to deal with a karmic cause in previous incarnations."[4] Our present state of physical and mental health is heavily influenced by past lives, so we should not be surprised if we cannot identify the causes of a specific illness by the use of modern medicine. As Steiner argues,

> in every incarnation there are certain prime causes which come into play from incarnation to incarnation, and these will be karmically balanced in the next life. When examining the next life we can observe the causes. If an accident happens, however, for which in spite of all means at our disposal we can find no causes in an earlier life, then we must conceive that this will be balanced in a later life. Karma is not fate. From every life something is carried into later lives.[5]

Diseases are not just an evil which we must get rid of by all means, but rather spiritual devices which direct us towards spiritual growth. This is the reason why Steiner rejected vaccination. He referred to the smallpox vaccination in particular as being counter-productive:

> If we destroy the susceptibility to smallpox, we are concentrating only on the external side of karmic activity. If on the one side we

---

1. Steiner and Wegman, *Fundamentals of Therapy*, 5.
2. Steiner and Wegman, *Fundamentals of Therapy*, 5.
3. Steiner and Wegman, *Fundamentals of Therapy*, 7.
4. Steiner, "Karma of the Higher Beings," online.
5. Steiner, "Karma of the Higher Beings."

go in for hygiene, it is necessary that on the other we should feel it our duty to contribute to the person whose organism has been so transformed, something also for the good of his soul.[6]

In other words, although vaccination could indeed prevent smallpox, it would hinder the spiritual healing of one's karma. A compromise could be reached and vaccination allowed, but only if followed by "spiritual education," that is, by being taught the anthroposophic worldview.

The other major difference from modern medicine is that human nature must be seen in a four-dimensional way. The view of human nature and healing promoted by AM is said to be holistic, for "to the knowledge of the *physical* man which alone is accessible to the natural-scientific methods of today, Anthroposophy adds that of *spiritual* man."[7]

The physical body, the one investigated and treated by modern medicine, is just one of four bodies which compose human nature. If we had only this physical body, it would decay immediately, because such a complex system cannot subsist by itself against the force of entropy. What keeps the physical body alive is the etheric body, which we share with plants. It is the equivalent of the vital sheath (the *pranamaya kosha*) we have met in Hinduism, the body that feeds the physical body with vital energy. If we had only the physical and the etheric body, we would be perpetually asleep, unable to feel anything. The body that makes us active and sensitive is the astral body (or the soul), which we share with animals. But unlike animals, human beings are conscious because they have a fourth body. This is the self (also called Ego or spirit), the component of our nature that makes us think about the meaning of life. It passes through many incarnations according to the law of karma, though not primarily as a punishment for ignorance or sins, but as the way to evolve to higher states of consciousness. In Steiner's words, the self "is the intelligent, rational soul. It is the indestructible individuality which can learn to build the other bodies – the 'inexpressible,' the human self and the divine self."[8]

This is, in short, how human nature is defined in anthroposophical medicine, and on this foundation is defined one's state of health or illness, as well as the necessary treatment. Health problems arise from our karma and the lack of balance between the four bodies. An illness is thus more than just the problem of the physical body, and the right diagnosis must

6. Steiner, "Karma of the Higher Beings."
7. Steiner and Wegman, *Fundamentals of Therapy*, 5.
8. Steiner, "An Esoteric Cosmology."

be reached after a careful observation of all the manifestations of the patient, both physical and mental, for they speak of the health of all the four bodies. Since modern medicine examines and treats only the physical and disregards the other three bodies, it is considered to be far less effective than AM.

In order to find out where the imbalance between the four bodies lies, and thus formulate the right treatment, it is vital to know the temperament of the patient. The four temperaments are the same as those defined in classical psychology (sanguine, phlegmatic, choleric, and melancholic), but according to AM they are produced by the prevalence of one of the four bodies. In the Choleric the self predominates; in the Sanguine the astral; in the Phlegmatic the etheric predominates, and in the Melancholic the physical body.[9]

Here in short is how AM correlates each temperament with the general health problems one develops: If the self is overactive the other bodies are underdeveloped. As a result, cholerics are generally less physically developed and thus shorter.[10] Sanguine people manifest a state of restlessness and agitation because of the domination of the astral body, which produces a more supple body and an elastic kind of walking. When the astral body gains absolute dominion over the others, it is no longer controlled by the self, and the self becomes too weak. This imbalance can be observed in the eyes: "Our eyes are held in place by the stable but delicate balance between the ego and the astral body. When a patient's eyes protrude to as if attempting to escape from the body, we know that the ego is too weak to keep them in their proper place."[11] The phlegmatic has a large body, either too tall or too fat, because the etheric body determines the outgrowth of the physical body. Therefore we find clues about the state of the etheric body by looking at one's bodily constitution. It will tell us how the etheric body influenced the growth of that individual in childhood, causing it to be too fast or too slow. The last of the four, the melancholic, is dominated by the physical body, and therefore the astral cannot control it effectively, which can be observed in the fact that he or she "has a drooping head (. . .) the glance is downwards, the eye sad."[12]

---

9. Steiner, *Medicine*, 63–67.
10. Steiner, *Medicine*, 80. Napoleon is given as a good example here.
11. Steiner, *Medicine*, 168.
12. Steiner, *Medicine*, 84–85.

Intense and frequent dreams indicate the excessive development of the self and of the astral body, to the disadvantage of the physical body.[13] If a person is active or rather slow, we find a clue about the mobility of the self and the astral body. In a slow person these two bodies remain active only at an unconscious level.[14] Even myopia indicates a dysfunctional relationship between the bodies, showing that a person has a self and astral body "reluctant to intervene in the physical body."[15] Mental disorders are not diseases of the self because the self "is always healthy and incapable of falling ill."[16] Their true origin lies in the fact that the self (the spirit) cannot manifest itself properly because of imbalances found between the other three bodies. Ita Wegman points out that,

> The primary factor in all psychiatric illnesses never lies in the upper part of the body, but always in the lower part, in the organs belonging to the four systems of the liver, kidneys, heart, and lungs. In the case of someone who is losing interest in outer life and beginning to brood and act out delusions, the most important concern is always to get an idea of the constitution of this person's pulmonary process.[17]

Following a similar intuition, "if we observe someone in whom obstinacy, pigheadedness, and self-righteousness appear, indicating a certain immobility or rigidity in thinking, this should lead us to investigate the status of liver function in the person in question."[18] It is because we wrongly locate the source of psychological problems in the head that modern psychiatry has such discouraging success rates.

This association between bodies, temperaments, organs, and diseases is "strange" only for practitioners of modern medicine. In anthroposophical medicine we find even more such profound associations, which go beyond those discussed above, to include the four bodies, four temperaments, four fundamental elements, and four cardinal organs. The four fundamental elements are the same as those we find in Hindu cosmology (fire, air, water, and earth), and the four cardinal organs of the physical body are the heart,

---

13. Steiner, *Medicine*, 180.
14. Steiner, *Medicine*, 180.
15. Steiner, *Medicine*, 181.
16. Steiner, *Medicine*, 158–59. In German they are called *Geisteskrankheiten* (diseases of the spirit).
17. Steiner, *Medicine*, 159–60.
18. Steiner, *Medicine*, 160.

kidneys, liver, and lungs. A deeper analysis of these connections would, however, go beyond the limits of this book.[19] Another part of AM treatment that I will omit in this chapter is the use of eurythmy, the anthroposophical art of movement, which is used both in Waldorf schools and in anthroposophical medicine. Although it is claimed to be an art expressed in movement and speech, and practitioners give the impression of doing a particular kind of gymnastics, eurythmy is a way of teaching anthroposophical concepts, of balancing the forces within the body and of getting in tune with the universe.

3.2 FOUR BODIES, SEVEN PLANETS, AND SEVEN HEALING METALS

As we have seen above, the self is the immortal element of human nature, the body that reincarnates. At death, the astral, etheric, and physical bodies are lost, and the self ascends into higher spiritual realms. When it descends to a new incarnation the three bodies are rebuilt. The forces of the self form the astral body, then the etheric, and ultimately the physical (during the nine months of pregnancy). The astral body bears this name because it is rebuilt as the self passes through seven astral domains corresponding to the seven planets of astrology, in the following order: Saturn, Jupiter, Mars, Sun, Venus, Mercury, and Moon.[20] To each planet is connected a metal, in the same order: lead, tin, iron, gold, copper, mercury, and silver.[21]

As the self crosses the seven astral spheres it rebuilds the astral body, and the qualities gathered in this "descent" are reflected in the functioning of the physical organs. For instance, passing through the planetary sphere of Saturn, the self receives the forces necessary for the formation of bones and of hematopoietic cells (in the bone marrow). Saturn is also the sphere where memory and self-consciousness are formed.[22] On this assumption, it is said that people who have difficulties in facing reality had an issue in the formation of consciousness when their self passed through the sphere of Saturn. These people must be treated with lead (the metal of Saturn).

---

19. Victor Bott, one of the founding fathers of AM, presents a long discussion of these relationships in his *Anthroposophische Medizin* [*Anthroposophical Medicine*].

20. Obviously, the sun and the moon are not planets, but here we follow the codification of astrology.

21. Bott, *Anthroposophische Medizin*, 30.

22. Bott, *Anthroposophische Medizin*, 35–39.

Specifically, to young girls who go about with their "head in the clouds," an ointment of lead salts must be applied over the spleen, because the spleen is the organ of Saturn and the region responsible for one's enthusiasm. The salt of a heavy metal would bring them down to earth.[23]

An example of how a corresponding metal, planet, and organ interact is the link between gold, the sun, and the heart. The heart corresponds to the center of the planetary system, that is, to the sun. This correspondence was formulated following the observation that the Sun has phases of physical expansion and contraction, in a similar way to the heart.[24] Therefore, when crossing the solar sphere, the astral body receives the forces necessary for the formation of the heart and the circulatory system. On this assumption, the metal that heals heart diseases is gold, the metal associated with the sun.

In order to grasp the complexity of theories at work in AM, let me present a particular case. In Ita Wegman's book, one of the successful cases is that of a 26-year-old woman who was in a state of restlessness and hyperactivity. From this condition it was assumed that the self did not have enough dominion over the astral body, which meant that the self could not impose its influence in order to calm the patient's state of anxiety. She also suffered from constipation, and this disruption of digestive activity was said to cause migraines and vomiting. In the morning, when waking up, she suffered from tachycardia (cardiac palpitations) and fear, which was triggered by the accumulation of carbon dioxide in the blood during the night. The AM diagnosis was that the astral body did not sufficiently control the etheric and physical bodies, which had caused growth retardation and frequent back pain. Given the intense dreams she had, it was obvious that the astral body had an intense activity when it found itself separated from the etheric and physical bodies. Taking all these clues into account, the treatment had to seek to weaken the astral body and strengthen the self. The recommended remedy for the self was copper, applied as ointment on the lumbar region, as well as minimal doses of lead (for the astral body), because "lead draws the astral body together and awakens in it the forces through which it unites more intensely with the physical body and the etheric."[25] As a result of this treatment, the patient was healed of her emotional liability, as well as of back pain, migraines, and constipation.

23. Bott, *Anthroposophische Medizin*, 39.
24. Bott, *Anthroposophische Medizin*, 72.
25. Steiner and Wegman, *Fundamentals of Therapy*, 44–45.

3.3 THE TREATMENT FOR CANCER

One of the most unusual treatments offered in AM is that of cancer. This fatal illness is said to appear because "in a part of the human body where there should be no internal sense organs formed the astral body suddenly begins to want to form sense organs there, to wake up and perceive things. The cancer is only something wishing to be ear or eye in a wrong place."[26] Generally speaking, "all tumor formations and carcinomas are really misplaced attempts to form a sense organ."[27]

The cause of this disturbance is that "the ego activity is not penetrating in the right way out of the etheric body."[28] In other words, the etheric body must be supported so that it might be "permeated by the ego and astral body."[29] According to AM there are centrifugal forces in the etheric body, "forces that want to move out into the cosmos," and cancer appears when "the astral body and ego are unable to counteract them sufficiently."[30] Given this situation, Steiner's intuition led him to think that "either we must attempt to strengthen the astral body by turning to the plant kingdom or we must suppress the effects of the etheric body by turning to the animal kingdom."[31] The choice was made for the first solution, and so the miraculous properties of mistletoe were discovered.

Steiner came up with the idea of using mistletoe intuitively, starting from the particular properties of this plant. Mistletoe is a parasitic plant with a vegetation cycle different from that of the host tree. It blooms in early spring, in summer it enjoys the shade of the tree that it lives off, and it remains green all winter. Since it slows down the development of the host tree above its attachment point, Steiner concluded that it takes away the power to grow vertically. This means that it defeats the etheric body of the tree, taking away its normal ability to conform itself to the centrifugal force which causes it to grow vertically.[32] This property of intervening against the normal course of tree development can be used when the *human* etheric

---

26. Steiner, *Medicine*, 119–20.
27. Steiner, *Medicine*, 174.
28. Steiner, *Medicine*, 133.
29. Steiner, *Medicine*, 133.
30. Steiner, *Medicine*, 169.
31. Steiner, *Medicine*, 133.
32. Steiner, *Medicine*, 151–52.

body becomes out of balance and causes the chaotic development of the physical body, which we see in cancer.

Another observation that formed Steiner's belief about the effectiveness of mistletoe in cancer treatment is that trees sometimes have tumors, swellings of the trunk that affect the development of the tree above that tumor. His interpretation was that such a tumor is the equivalent of a situation in which the tree would become a parasite of itself, following the disruption of the etheric body. As a result, its development will take place beneath the tumor, downwards, not upwards, as normal. Mistletoe has the same effect on the tree, for it prevents it from developing upwards by weakening its etheric body. The medical application is that this effect can be transferred to the human body affected by cancer, which induces a similar disorder. The etheric body of the cancer patient is too strong, and mistletoe can extract some of that excessive power, as it does in the case of a tree. In practice, for the weakening and resorption of the cancerous tumor mistletoe extract (Iscador) injections are given around the tumor, in order to weaken the etheric body.[33] If the mistletoe extract is mixed with silver salts, it becomes more effective for abdominal cancers, because silver is a heavy metal and moves the beneficial action of mistletoe towards the abdomen.[34]

Continuing with his observations and insights on the unique development of some plants, Steiner concluded that Christmas rose (*Helleborus niger*) must also have special properties, for it blooms in winter. Its use would be more appropriate for tumors in men. Why a differentiated treatment by gender? Mistletoe grows in trees, while Christmas rose grows on the ground. The plant that grows on the ground would be more appropriate for treating men's tumors because men are "more closely related to earthly factors," that is, they are more pragmatic, realistic and down-to-earth. Women are "more closely related to supra-earthly factors," so for them mistletoe, which grows in trees, is more beneficial.[35]

3.4 THE SPIRITUAL EVOLUTION OF HUMANKIND

Anthroposophical medicine must be understood in a wider context than the need for balancing the four bodies and the connections between bodies, organs, fundamental elements, planets, and metals. This wider context is

33. Steiner, *Medicine*, 170–71.
34. Steiner, *Medicine*, 155.
35. Steiner, *Medicine*, 157.

the perpetual spiritual evolution of humankind and the need to understand which stage we are now at in this evolution. Victor Bott argues that the anthroposophical view of human evolution is much broader than that of Darwinism:

> Rudolf Steiner opened the path of spiritual investigation to reveal the whole process, and to show that the discoveries of paleontology are in fact only material evidence of a wider evolutionary process, whose impulse can be found only in a spiritual dimension.[36]

Anthroposophy teaches that the evolution of our world has a spiritual ground. It is not the mineral world that generates life, following a process of random biochemical reactions (as in Darwinism), because the spiritual world *pre-exists* the physical world. It is the spiritual world that pushes the physical into higher forms of organization. In Bott's words, "beings existed before the mineral kingdom" because "these beings first existed spiritually" and their physical existence "is the result of a process of condensation into a material form."[37]

This perpetual spiritual evolution of our world is the proper context in which we must understand the destiny of humankind and its connection to the nature and aim of anthroposophical medicine. In this section I will provide only a brief introduction to the way Steiner defines his view of the perpetual spiritual evolution of human beings,[38] in order to understand, if it is not yet sufficiently clear, to what extent it is compatible with Christianity. Instead of using many references from Steiner's books, it will be sufficient to mention what he said in a single conference, entitled "The Cosmic Ego and the Human Ego. The Nature of Christ the Resurrected."[39] This source alone will provide enough information to understand the relationship between anthroposophy and Christianity.

At its present stage of evolution, human nature is made up of the four bodies mentioned so far in this chapter. From this stage we will evolve

---

36. Bott, *Anthroposophische Medizin*, 14.

37. Bott, *Anthroposophische Medizin*, 15.

38. Given the limitations of this book, I cannot explore Steiner's philosophy more deeply. This topic is worth analyzing, at least for those interested in understanding the ground of the Waldorf school movement, and especially for those who entrust their children to this kind of education. Christians interested in learning about this side of anthroposophy can get in touch with a network of former Waldorf parents and teachers called "People for Legal and Non-Sectarian Schools (PLANS)" at waldorfcritics.org.

39. Steiner, "Cosmic Ego and Human Ego." All further quotations in this section are from this conference.

further, acquiring new spiritual bodies. In the next stages of our evolution we will acquire the fifth (the Spirit-Self), the sixth (the Life-Spirit), and the seventh body (the Spirit-Man). There are many other beings in the spiritual universe who already have these seven bodies, following many incarnations on Earth, on the Moon, Sun, and Saturn. They are called archangels. Another kind of spiritual beings are those who have not followed the right path in spiritual evolution and, as a result, are not yet at the level they should have reached long ago. They are called "Luciferic beings." This name should not scare us. By virtue of the perpetual evolution of all beings, anthroposophy does not admit the possibility of existing eternally damned beings, as are demons in Christianity. Luciferic beings are those who have stopped developing while having reached their fifth, sixth or seventh body. They no longer have a physical body, because having a physical body is only possible up to the human stage, that is, until they are in the process of perfecting their fourth body, the self. Therefore, for these beings the only possibility to continue their evolution is to find a "substitute physical body," which means that they need the help of the most evolved beings that still retain a physical body. In other words, in order to continue their evolution, the Luciferic beings need us, humans.

The geniuses of humanity, the great heroes, the founders of cities, and leaders of great nations were people "*possessed* by higher Luciferic beings." In Steiner's words, "Luciferic beings always had the longing to continue their evolution in the way described, by possessing human beings; and *they are still doing that today*." The relationship between the possessed humans and the Luciferic spirits is one of symbiosis. They help us and we help them to evolve. On the one hand, "these Luciferic beings take us and develop *themselves in us*," and on the other hand, through the intercession of these spirits, we reach the formation of the fifth and sixth body.

According to Steiner's philosophy, such teachings should not scare us. On the contrary, we should rejoice for having the privilege of evolving, because being possessed leads us to higher levels of spirituality and transforms us into geniuses. In Steiner's words, "the Luciferic spirits are absolutely necessary, and the gifted men of earth are they in whom the Luciferic spirit is working diligently." From here we can assume that Steiner was himself such a genius, a possessed man in whom a superior being was at work, to raise both him and his followers to higher spiritual realms. One of these spirits is plainly called Lucifer, and to him must be "assigned a share in the great cultural progress of the earth." The attitude of Christians, who know well who Lucifer is, what possession is and what kind of spirits it involves, is ridiculed. Steiner states that it is only the narrow-mindedness of Christians that makes them "see in the Luciferic being only the wicked devil." Therefore, his urge is that we "must free ourselves from narrowness, from all orthodox Christianity which calls Lucifer only a devil worthy of hatred."

So here we find expressed the goal and climax of anthroposophy! Not only does it teach the pre-existence of the soul, karma, and reincarnation, but it goes much further. True wisdom and spiritual evolution is achieved by being possessed by Luciferic beings! Can there still be any doubt on the true spiritual direction to which anthroposophy invites us?[40] Even Steiner was aware that these beings are what "traditional Christians" call "demons." On this issue he was right. Therefore faithful Christians should stay away from anthroposophy and its many applications, including AM.

---

40. In the same conference, as in all the rest, he denies many other fundamental Christian teachings. Christ is only a spiritual teacher who evolved spiritually just like us, but in a different realm. The man who died on the cross was the *human* Jesus, whose body disintegrated in the tomb, and was seen afterwards as "an etheric body, condensed to visibility by the Christ force." These views are a flat denial of Christian doctrine, following a Gnostic interpretation of Jesus Christ's identity.

4

Ayurveda

THIS ANCIENT FORM OF alternative medicine has its origin in India, and its name means "the science of life."[1] My assessment of Ayurveda will follow the guidelines laid down by two of its most popular representatives, Deepak Chopra and Vasant Lad. Chopra is a best-selling author, public speaker, promoter of Ayurveda since 1984, and one of the best known voices of the New Age movement.[2] Lad, the other major advocate of Ayurveda in the U.S. since 1979, is the author of many books and the founder of the Ayurvedic Institute in Santa Fe, New Mexico, as well as a member of other Ayurvedic establishments in the U.S.[3]

4.1 AYURVEDIC TYPOLOGY

Like other forms of alternative medicine, Ayurveda claims that it does not treat diseases, but persons, each with his or her own individual traits. Ayurvedic typology works on the assumption that our individual constitution is produced by the combination of three factors, called *doshas*: *vata*, *pitta*, and *kapha*. The proportion in which the three *doshas* participate in

---

1. In Sanskrit *Ayus* means *life*, and *Veda* means *knowledge*.

2. Among his many top positions in promoting Ayurveda, he was the director of the Maharishi Ayurveda Health Center for Stress Management, founding president of Maharishi Ayur-Veda Products International, Inc (MAPI), president of the American Association of Ayurvedic Medicine, and co-founder of the Chopra Center for Wellbeing.

3. Here you can read the story of his initiation and success in the U.S.: https://www.ayurveda.com/about/about-vasant-lad (retrieved December 13, 2019).

one's constitution determines seven types of individuals, with particular likes and dislikes, psychological preferences, and physical characteristics. Each type has a distinctive set of physical and psychological traits, an optimal diet, and a recommended lifestyle.[4] The first three types are given by the absolute dominance of one *dosha*, the next three are defined by the contribution of two *doshas* (one principal, the other secondary), and in the seventh type all three *doshas* bear a similar influence.

In their turn, the *doshas* are generated by the five fundamental elements of Hindu cosmology (ether, air, fire, water, and earth). To each element corresponds a sense organ (ear, skin, eye, tongue, and nose), its sense (hearing, touch, sight, taste, and smell), a kind of action (speech, apprehension, walking, procreation, and excretion), and an organ of that action (tongue, hand, foot, genitals, and anus).[5]

Vata is the factor that determines movement, breathing, blood circulation, the nervous system, and emotional factors such as anxiety, vigor, and fear. *Pitta* determines metabolism, food, air, and water processing, as well as anger, hate, and jealousy. *Kapha* is the factor which controls the body's shape and structure and forms the tissues, but also controls body resistance and perseverance.[6]

As long as the *doshas* are balanced, the individual is healthy and happy, but when they get out of balance, all kinds of problems appear. For instance, when *pitta* gets out of balance, one becomes very critical and angry, while the physical body develops gastric hyperacidity, diarrhea, and various skin diseases. The imbalance of *vata* generates anxiety and fear, associated with constipation, arthritis, and insomnia. *Kapha* out of balance generates excessive attachments, depression, bronchitis, and allergies.[7]

4.2 DIAGNOSIS AND TREATMENT IN AYURVEDA

Once the individual type has been established, by using a questionnaire and a long interview, the practitioner proceeds to determine the patient's present state (*vikruti*), the extent to which the *doshas* are in balance for that given type. This requires a long and elaborate process of observation, which is quite different from that of modern medicine, as Ayurveda examines

---

4. Chopra, *Perfect Health*, 32–33.
5. Lad, *Ayurveda*, 23–25.
6. Chopra, *Perfect Health*, 25–26, Lad, *Ayurveda*, 29–30.
7. Lad, *The Complete Book*, 2.

Ayurveda

pulses, the tongue, face, mouth, skin, fingers, and nails of the patient, for each provides unique indications of one's health.

Pulses are taken above the wrist of both hands of the patient by using three fingers—the index, the middle and the ring finger—separately. Pulse examination means measuring not the heart rate, but the balance of the *doshas* and the health of internal organs. Each *dosha* has its own pulse and a particular nature: that of the *vata* is perceived as the movement of a snake, that of the *pitta* as the jump of a frog, while that of the *kapha* resembles the floating of a swan.[8] Each finger senses the pulse corresponding to a certain internal organ, twelve in total, since there is both a deep and a superficial pulse sensed by each of the six fingers of the Ayurvedic practitioner.[9]

The tongue provides information on one's health by its size, color, shape, contour, edges, and coatings. The state of several internal organs can be read in different parts of the surface of the tongue. The heart is represented between the tip and the middle of the tongue, lungs on the margins, and the stomach in the middle, with the spleen and the liver on its sides, the intestines in the back part and the kidneys on the sides. If there are some blemishes, deposits, swellings or depressions on these areas, the corresponding organs are not well.[10] On the lips can be read complementary information about these organs. For instance, the lower lip shows the condition of the intestines, and the corners of the mouth the status of the kidneys.[11]

The face is said to be the mirror of the mind. Even wrinkles give precious insights about the patient's mental state. For instance, horizontal wrinkles on the forehead betray deep worries. As Lad points out, "a vertical line between the eyebrows on the right side indicates your emotions are repressed in the liver," or in the spleen, if the line is closer to the left eyebrow.[12] The shape of the eyes indicates the dominant *dosha*, while internal organs and their diseases are represented on different parts of the eye. Fingers also correspond to internal organs. The thumb shows the state of the brain, the index that of the lungs, the middle the condition of the small intestine, the

---

8. Lad, *Ayurveda*, 54.

9. The twelve organs assessed by pulse examination are: heart, small intestine, spleen, stomach, kidneys, bladder, lungs, large intestine, liver, gallbladder, equilibrium of the three *doshas* (obviously not an organ) and pericardium. We will encounter a similar pattern in acupuncture.

10. Lad, *Ayurveda*, 60–62.

11. Lad, *Ayurveda*, 65.

12. Lad, *Ayurveda*, 62–64.

ring finger indicates problems of the kidneys, and the little finger points to the state of the heart.[13]

The lack of balance between the three *doshas* causes the buildup of toxins (*ama*), of both a physical and an emotional nature. There are five ways to eliminate these toxins, called the "five actions" (*pancha karma*): therapeutic vomiting, purgation, enema, nasal administration of medication, and bloodletting. Vomiting is used to cleanse the lungs of mucus and consequently to balance the *kapha dosha*. As Lad argues, therapeutic vomiting is also indicated for skin diseases, chronic asthma, diabetes, chronic indigestion, edema, epilepsy, and tonsillitis.[14] Purgations are used to remove toxins from the blood and clean the *pitta dosha*. Laxatives can treat skin diseases, chronic fever, abdominal tumors, intestinal worms, and gout.[15] Enemas are used to treat *vata* imbalance, manifested as constipation, chronic fever, sexual dysfunction, kidney stones, heart and colon pain, and gastric hyperacidity.[16] Nasal cleaning is required for head, nose, eye, and ear diseases, on the assumption that the nose is the closest external orifice to these organs. Bloodletting is used to treat urticaria, eczema, acne, and other skin diseases, as well as cases of swelled liver or spleen.[17]

Besides these five methods of eliminating toxins, a crucial factor for health is diet, which must be appropriate to one's type. The diet should take into account incompatibilities between foods and how they strengthen or weaken the influence of a particular *dosha*.

Another important influence on health is formulated by Ayurvedic astrology. For example, Mars influences the health of blood and liver, Saturn that of the muscles, Venus of sexual organs, and Mercury that of the mind.[18]

As we can see so far, Ayurveda has a very different view of diagnosis and treatment from modern medicine. Since this book is not a comparison of Western and Eastern traditions in medicine, nor about the medical efficiency of its remedies, in the remaining part of this chapter we will investigate the deeper spiritual direction to which Ayurveda leads, which should be quite distressing and even alarming for Christians.

---

13. Lad, *Ayurveda*, 65–67.

14. Lad, *Ayurveda*, 70.

15. Lad, *Ayurveda*, 72–73. One of the laxatives used in Ayurveda is one's own urine (Lad, *Ayurveda*, 44).

16. Lad, *Ayurveda*, 75.

17. Lad, *Ayurveda*, 78.

18. Lad, *Ayurveda*, 107.

4.3 AYURVEDA AND ITS SPIRITUAL TEACHINGS

It is not wrong for a Christian to know his or her temperament, to use questionnaires to identify personal strengths and weaknesses, to follow a healthy diet, and take outdoor exercise. Having a balanced lifestyle and avoiding stress is, or should be, recommended by every family doctor. Herbal remedies of the Himalayas could also be of help, although they must first be tested according to the standards of medical science. However, Ayurveda is much more than the use of herbal remedies and the urge to follow a healthy lifestyle.

The harmless recommendations on diet and physical exercise are accompanied by Hindu meditation and Yoga, and along with finding the balance between the three *doshas*, Ayurveda requires finding the right balance between the physical body, the mind, and the self (*atman*). This makes Ayurveda a subtle bridge from utilizing a nature-friendly medicine to adopting a Hindu worldview. Although Christians may be happy to find that the ultimate purpose of Ayurveda is to know "the Creator," a closer look will show that the "Creator" meant by Lad is "Cosmic Consciousness," which is another name for Brahman.[19] Therefore we are not dealing with a mere ancient nature-friendly therapy, but, in Lad's words, with "a profound science of living that encompasses the whole of life and relates the life of the individual to the life of the universe."[20]

Beyond harmless requirements for balancing the *vata dosha* such as having regular habits, seeking silence, drinking liquids, avoiding stress, resting, and restrained eating,[21] we are told by Chopra that "the best rest, aside from sleep, is the deep relaxation provided by meditation."[22] This is not any kind of meditation, but Transcendental Meditation (in short, TM).[23] Chopra affirms that he has been attracted to the practice of TM since the 1970s for two reasons. One was the desire to grow spiritually and reach "an expanded state of mental and spiritual development," and the other was scientific studies that have allegedly proven the medical benefits of Hindu meditation.[24] As a follower and former disciple of Maharishi Mahesh Yogi

---

19. Lad, *The Complete Book*, 3.
20. Lad, *Ayurveda*, 1.
21. Chopra, *Perfect Health*, 95.
22. Chopra, *Perfect Health*, 96.
23. Chopra, *Perfect Health*, 96.
24. Chopra, *Perfect Health*, 124.

(1918–2008), the founder of TM, Chopra cannot help recommending this practice to those who want "perfect health," as the title of one of his most popular books says, for it is considered the best help "to integrate the mind-body link."[25]

Due to the close association between Chopra's use of Ayurveda and Transcendental Meditation,[26] we need to remember some important facts about this movement. It was founded by the Indian guru Maharishi Mahesh to promote a form of Hindu meditation suitable for the secularized Western world. Mahesh was able to present Hindu concepts in an attractive form for Westerners, invoking scientific evidence for the benefits of meditation on health. Using pseudo-scientific language, he even managed to fool the American educational system into introducing TM into public high schools. Soon its religious character was revealed, and TM programs in schools were shut down. Here is a short fragment from the initiation ceremony, which speaks for itself:

> Guru in the glory of Brahma, Guru in the glory of Vishnu, Guru in the glory of the great Lord Shiva, Guru in the glory of the personified transcendental fullness of Brahman, to Him, to Shri Guru Dev adorned with glory, I bow down.[27]

In TM the synonym used for Brahman is simply *Being*. Mahesh affirmed it as "the ultimate reality of all that exists, lives, or is (. . .) of all that was, is or will be, (. . .) the eternal and unbounded, the basis of all the phenomenal existence of the cosmic life."[28] Using a typical pantheistic illustration, Being is the "unbounded ocean of pure consciousness," while the individual is "the expression of cosmic life, just as a wave is the expression of the ocean."[29] We come into existence as a result of karma generated in earlier lives, while liberation from karma and reincarnation, as the

---

25. Chopra, *Perfect Health*, 96.

26. Chopra met Mahesh in 1984, and then became the main voice in the U.S. for promoting Ayurveda as a holistic path to well-being. As a result, in 1989, Mahesh conferred on him the title of "Dhanvantari of heaven and earth" (Dhanvantari means "the doctor of gods") (Stewart et al., *Basic Questions*, 46).

27. You can find the whole text of the initiation ceremony at http://minet.org/www.trancenet.net/secrets/puja/tradt.shtml. For more information on TM see http://tmfree.blogspot.com/.

28. Mahesh, *The Science of Being*, 21

29. Mahesh, *The Science of Being*, 69. From this we can better understand what Chopra means by quoting a Vedic verse, which says that "we are ripples in the ocean of consciousness" (Chopra, *Perfect Health*, 313).

Ayurveda

Upanishads also assert, is achieved through defeating ignorance and knowing our true nature.

The actual practice of TM requires repeating a mantra for 20 minutes, twice a day. The mantra is a word of one or two syllables, allegedly suited to each individual practitioner, but in fact the same for all of the same age and same sex. Although TM teachers claim that mantras are simple sounds that produce a mental effect, or create the right "vibration" in our mind, in an early writing Mahesh makes it clear that mantras are more than that:

> Thus we find that any sound can serve our purpose of training the mind to become sharp. But we do not select any sound like "mike," flower, table, pen, wall etc. because such ordinary sounds can do nothing more than merely sharpening the mind; whereas there are some special sounds which have the additional efficacy of producing vibrations whose effects are found to be congenial to our way of life. This is the scientific reason why we do not select any word at random. For our practice we select only the suitable mantras of personal Gods. Such mantras fetch to us the grace of personal Gods and make us happier in every walk of life.[30]

Therefore the repetition of mantras has nothing to do with science, but is rather a way of invoking a Hindu god, and thus a form of Hindu devotion. This being the nature and role of mantras, we realize that their use is intended to enhance the inner powers of human beings by invoking the power of a particular god, the patron of that mantra. As such, the practice of TM is not a simple self-help technique that anybody can learn from books. One must follow it as religious tradition that teaches specific rules on how to tap into spiritual resources. Chopra demands that one should learn it from "a qualified instructor,"[31] that is, a guru in the tradition of TM.

The start of one's proper practice of TM is, as in any other Hindu sect, a ritual called initiation. A similar religious ritual is performed in Hindu temples when one is consecrated as a devotee of a particular Hindu god, in front of his or her sacred image or statue. The initiation ritual in TM takes place before the image of Guru Dev, the Indian guru who initiated Mahesh and sent him as a missionary to spread this meditation method throughout the world.

In a similar way to TM, Ayurveda as "medicine" is aimed at helping us achieve a deeper vision of reality, which is that of pantheistic Hinduism.

---

30. Mahesh, *Beacon Light Of The Himalayas*, online.
31. Chopra, *Perfect Health*, 130.

Chopra invites us to realize that "we are simply localized concentrations of energy and intelligence in the universal field,"[32] and suggests we should do Yoga exercises (called "fun exercises") in order to "enliven the connection between our inner and outer worlds."[33] It follows the same vision we have met in the previous chapter, formulated by the sages of Hinduism, who "proclaimed that the purpose of attending to the body is to support the state of being known as enlightenment." [34] Thus Chopra leads us to the same goal, that is, to the union of self (*atman*) with its primordial source (Brahman), in a state in which we understand that we are "unbounded beings temporarily masquerading as individuals" and that "the knower, the process of knowing, and that which is known are one and the same."[35] This is the "state of perfect health," formulated in Ayurvedic terms.[36]

Therefore to affirm that meditation is "a purely mechanical technique employed for twenty minutes morning and evening," and that the mantra is entrusted "not for its meaning but strictly for its sound" for it "attracts the mind and leads it, effortlessly and naturally, to a slightly subtler level of the thinking process,"[37] is a gross distortion of a religious reality, which can have medical benefits only as a secondary effect. Meditation is part of a Hindu religious practice and has the same goal as Yoga, "to seek still subtler levels of thought until eventually all thought is left behind."[38] Those "subtler" levels are the upper stages of Yoga practice, aimed at bringing the mind under control in order to achieve the liberation of the self.

4.4 OTHER HINDU PRACTICES IN AYURVEDA

Ayurveda promotes other elements of Hinduism as well. A particular recommended meditation is the one on breathing, which can be associated

---

32. Chopra, *Boundless Energy*, 5.
33. Chopra, *Perfect Health*, in the edition issued by Three Rivers, 2000, 5–6.
34. Chopra, *Perfect Health*, 6.
35. Chopra, *Perfect Health*, 6.
36. Vasant Lad, in his turn, confirms that Ayurveda is fully integrated into the Hindu worldview. He argues that the goal of life is to experience Cosmic Consciousness (another name for Brahman), which is achieved by harmonizing the four fundamental aspects of life: *dharma* (social and family duty), *artha* (professional success and wealth), *kama* (pleasures of life) and *moksha* (liberation of the self) (Lad, *The Complete Book*, 3).
37. Chopra, *Perfect Health*, 125.
38. Chopra, *Perfect Health*, 125.

with the "*so hum*" mantra.[39] Like any other mantra, it does not represent just two random syllables, but has a profound spiritual significance. "*So hum*" means "I am that reality"; that is, my inner self (*atman*) is of the same nature as the Supreme Self (Brahman). The equivalent of this mantra is one of the oldest formulas of the Upanishads, *Tat Tvam Asi* ("Thou are that"). Both are recommended by Chopra.[40] Brahman is hidden under the name of "superfield," "unified field," or "the ultimate reality that underlies all of nature,"[41] and the need to restore the *atman*-Brahman unity is formulated by the requirement to see ourselves as "part of the unified field" which "is in and around us all the time."[42]

Even Ayurvedic herbal therapy needs to be understood in spiritual terms. Chopra argues that in Ayurvedic medicine "herbs do not have the gross effect on the body that Western medicines do." [43] An Ayurvedic phytotherapist must know that Ayurvedic herbal remedies "introduce a subtle signal in the physiology – they 'talk' to the *doshas* and directly influence the flow of inner intelligence."[44]

Another important aspect of Ayurvedic therapy is the practice of physical exercise in order to increase vitality. It does not mean any kind of exercise, but executing specific Hatha Yoga *asanas*. As Lad affirms, "Ayurveda and yoga are sister sciences. (. . .) Yoga is the science of union with the Ultimate Being. Ayurveda is the science of living, of daily life."[45] A favorite cycle of *asanas* recommended by Chopra is the *Sun Salutation* (*Surya Namaskar*).[46] This is a very ancient practice in Hinduism, being mentioned as early as in the Vedic hymns, the earliest writings of Hinduism, in which it is a series of mantras recited in honor of the sun god (Surya). Yoga took

---

39. According to Lad there is a close link between breath and mind: "When breath stops, mind stops, because mind is the movement of breath" (*The Complete Book*, 78). If this meditation is done properly, it "leads to the union of the individual with the universal Cosmic Consciousness" (*The Complete Book*, 79; *Ayurveda*, 126).

40. Chopra, "I Am That," online.

41. Chopra, *Perfect Health*, 132.

42. Chopra, *Perfect Health*, 132.

43. Chopra, *Perfect Health*, 179.

44. Chopra, *Perfect Health*, 179.

45. Lad, *Ayurveda*, 113.

46. Chopra, *Perfect Health*, 268–77. Lad argues that the *Sun Salutation* is beneficial for the *vata* type, while the *Moon Salutation* (*Chandra Namaskar*) for the *pitta* type (Lad, *The Complete Book*, 60–61).

this practice and transformed it into a series of *asanas*, to which Western practitioners no longer associate the requested mantras.⁴⁷

A further technique borrowed from Hatha Yoga is breath control (*pranayama*). Chopra recommends breathing alternatively through the two nostrils, inspiring through one and exhaling through the other. He fails to recall the reason for doing so, which is the flux of *prana* through the *ida* and *pingala nadis*, adjacent to the *sushumna* central channel. Chopra presents *pranayama* as "the best prelude to meditation, since it effortlessly focuses your attention inward."⁴⁸ Lad, in his turn, explains that breathing alternately through the two nostrils leads to the balancing of masculine and feminine energy, and as a result, "when these energies are balanced, the neutral energy is awakened and one experiences pure awareness, which is called *brahman*."⁴⁹ Therefore Ayurvedic breathing control is part of a spiritual practice of self-discovery, not just a more efficient way of oxygenating the body.

Lad adds to these practices other therapeutic elements, such as the use of metals, crystals, color therapy, and aromatherapy. Certain metals can transfer their healing properties if they are boiled for a long time in water, which must then be drunk, on the grounds that "pure metals emit an astral light that provides a powerful counteraction to the negative pull of the planets."⁵⁰ For instance, water in which gold has been boiled is good for strengthening the heart and mind, while "copper-water" is a good tonic for the liver, the spleen and the lymphatic system, and "iron-water" is good for anemia.⁵¹ Precious and semiprecious stones attract the healing energies of planets,⁵² and colors are said to have inherent healing properties that can be transmitted to the patient directly or by drinking water which has been exposed to a certain color. For example, blue balances the *pitta dosha*,

---

47. For an introduction to the original meaning of Sun Salutation see https://yogainternational.com/article/view/the-ancient-origins-of-surya-namaskar-sun-salutation (retrieved December 16, 2019). For a brief presentation of the *asanas* used in Sun Salutation, breathing techniques, and the associated mantras see: https://en.wikipedia.org/wiki/Surya_Namaskara (retrieved March 1, 2019).

48. Chopra, *Perfect Health*, 298.

49. Lad, *The Complete Book*, 72. After describing the practice of *pranayama*, Lad urges readers to continue with the higher levels of Yoga practice, concentration, and meditation (Lad, *The Complete Book*, 76–78).

50. Lad, *Ayurveda*, 142.

51. Lad, *The Complete Book*, 276.

52. Lad, *The Complete Book*, 277–80.

Ayurveda

has a calming effect on the mind, and corrects liver dysfunctions.[53] And if a glass of water is wrapped in red paper and left in the sun for four hours, the red color will give the water the property to stimulate the formation of erythrocytes and stimulate circulation.[54]

4.5 AYURVEDA AND QUANTUM PHYSICS

As a novelty in endorsing a form of alternative medicine, Chopra attempts to prove the validity of Hindu teachings about the unity of the world in Brahman by recourse to quantum physics. In his words, "Maharishi Ayurveda, seen in its larger context, is nothing less than a technology for contacting the quantum level inside ourselves."[55] Since it reveals that energy is the basis of all physical, chemical, and biological phenomena, and that matter itself can be seen as condensed energy, Chopra argues that we could find in quantum physics a confirmation of the Hindu view of the unity of all existing things in Brahman. Insofar as, according to quantum physics, energy forms all things and phenomena, we could see in this energy-matter equivalence a correspondence to the Hindu view that Brahman generates all matter and beings. Another alleged application of quantum physics is intended to adapt the theory of the three bodies in Hinduism. As unseen energy is the basis of our seen world, Chopra upholds the existence of a subtle body in human nature, arguing that there is "a quantum pulse underlying your physical one, and a quantum heart beating it out. In fact Maharishi Ayurveda holds that all the organs and processes in your body have a quantum equivalent."[56]

Probably few of Chopra's readers understand what he means by such "quantum" language and think that he probably handles complicated scientific issues that confirm his spiritual approach. However, his attempt to provide a scientific aura to the spiritual bodies of Hinduism and to uphold a pantheistic worldview by the use of quantum physics is hardly convincing. A closer look reveals that Chopra's use of quantum physics is just a way of fooling those who have no clue as to what it really is,[57] a way of suggesting

---

53. Lad, *The Complete Book*, 282.
54. Lad, *Ayurveda*, 149.
55. Chopra, *Perfect Health*, 10.
56. Chopra, *Perfect Health*, 7.
57. We can observe the improper use of quantum physics when he says that atoms "are made up of subatomic particles—protons, neutrons, and electrons—which whirl

that in the mysterious world of subatomic particles we find a confirmation of the Hindu worldview and also a proof for the insufficiency of a materialistic worldview. He states:

> From the point of view of quantum physics, there is not much difference between fluctuations of thought arising within the unified field and the wave vibrations that give rise to the particles that make up the human body. In short, your thoughts are quantum events, subtle vibrations of the field, that have a profound influence on all the functions of your body.[58]

In other words, quantum physics would explain both the mental and the physical aspect of human nature and be their meeting point. However, his attempt neither confirms pantheism, nor defeats materialism. The world of subatomic particles and the concept that all matter can be reduced to energy does not confirm that mental phenomena have a material, or quantum, nature. Pantheism includes all phenomena, physical and mental, as manifestations of *one* reality, that of Brahman, while materialism cannot explain mental phenomena in physical terms. No matter how subtle the level at which we analyze subatomic particles, mental phenomena cannot have a material nature, and thus Chopra cannot succeed in explaining mental phenomena in physical terms, regardless of how much he strives to adapt quantum physics to his teachings. The mind (or the soul) is not of a material nature, so it cannot be represented under the categories of quantum physics, not even in the form of "wave vibrations that give rise to the particles that make up the human body."[59] The attempt to represent the mind as a physical mechanism is precisely the goal of a materialist worldview, and therefore to subscribe to this project would make one a follower of a materialistic worldview, against Chopra's struggle to prove it insufficient.

4.6 AYURVEDA AND CHRISTIANITY

Although it is presented as a healing method inspired by the ancient wisdom of India and "an art of daily living in harmony with the laws of

---

around each other at lightning speeds" (Chopra, *Boundless Energy*, 5). For more information on Chopra's use and abuse of quantum physics, see Stenger, "Quantum Quackery," online.

58. Chopra, *Boundless Energy*, 6–7.
59. Chopra, *Boundless Energy*, 7.

Ayurveda

nature,"[60] Ayurveda is in fact a subtle invitation to follow a Hindu worldview. Even if its herbal remedies can be beneficial, along with diet, massage, and tranquility, in Ayurveda they are just the starting point of a path that leads to adopting religious views alien to Christianity. The one who uses Ayurvedic therapy is led to experience Hindu meditation and Yoga, to be fully integrated into the universe, not as a special creature of God, but only as the wave in the ocean. This path is wholly alien to Christianity, for we are meant to know God and worship him forever as persons redeemed by grace. As Christians, our goal is not to break the bond of karma and attain an impersonal union with the universe, but to be free from the bondage of sin and enjoy full salvation, the state of a perfected relationship with God. This is absurd for Chopra, since in his view any traditional form of belief in God expresses an inability to overcome spiritual immaturity:

> I think religions fell back on personalizing the soul as "mine" or "yours" because just as an infinite God boggles the mind, so does the unbounded soul. Something more manageable was needed. Hence a personal God who sits above the clouds and looks down on his children, to whom he has provided a personal soul that fits neatly inside the heart. (. . .) The unbounded soul can't be lost or saved, it can't be denied or evicted by God, because God is made of the same pure awareness.[61]

In Chopra's view, happiness does not mean living in sanctifying grace, but the discovery of *atman*, "the unchanging essence of your inner self, your source."[62] One that has attained this knowledge is not afraid of death, for the simple reason that the self reincarnates and cannot "die." In his words, to the question "What happens to me when I die?" he answers: "Nothing happens, because I do not die."[63] No matter what happens, Chopra urges us to remember the law of karma:

> Remind yourself, *I am neither superior nor inferior to anyone who exists. Saint or sinner, the spirit that resides within me is the divine spirit. It has taken on a certain role in this lifetime, it has taken on other roles in other lifetimes. I honor the divine spirit in myself and in all beings as holy and sacred no matter what role it is playing.*[64]

60. Lad, *The Complete Book*, 1.
61. Chopra, *Reinventing the Body*, 172.
62. Chopra, *Power, Freedom and Grace*, 102.
63. Chopra, *Power, Freedom and Grace*, 62.
64. Chopra, *Power, Freedom and Grace*, 178.

The law of karma affirms an eternal return of the self to new lives, so the idea of death followed by a final judgment should not worry anyone.[65] Spiritual perfection means reaching what he calls "stage seven" of spiritual evolution. For one who has reached this stage, the answer to the question "Who are you?," can only be: "I am."[66] In order to dispel any doubts on what he means by these words, Chopra affirms that it is "the very answer that Jehovah gave Moses in the book of Exodus when he spoke from the burning bush"[67] In Chopra's view this is the highest level of *human* spiritual evolution. But for a Christian, such a vision can only be seen as the highest level of heresy, for no one and nothing except the persons of the Holy Trinity can assert inherent existence. A Christian can never say "I am" with the above meaning without breaking the First Commandment and thus committing a grave sin.

---

65. In his words, "Cause and effect never ends; its entanglement is so overwhelming that you could not end even a portion of your personal karma" (Chopra, *How to Know God*, 256–57).

66. Chopra, *How to Know God*, 275.

67. Chopra, *How to Know God*, 275–76.

5

Reiki

THE REIKI HEALING TECHNIQUE was discovered by the Japanese Buddhist monk Mikao Usui (1865–1926), while he was practicing Qigong on Mount Kurama, near Kyoto. It is said that in 1922 he had a mystical experience in which a "great and powerful spiritual light entered the top of his head"[1] and thus received an inexhaustible power that he had not known in Qigong. Reiki was then established as a new healing method by recourse to the universal *Chi* energy (*Ki*, in Japanese), and also as a path to spiritual perfection. The first school was founded in Japan by Usui himself, bearing the name Usui Reiki Ryoho Gakkai (Usui Reiki Healing Method Learning Society). In the Western world Reiki was introduced by Hawayo Takata, a Japanese-born American, who learned it from one of Usui's disciples (Chujiro Hayashi) after she was herself healed through Reiki.

Takata spread the false information that Usui was a Christian priest and the president of a Christian university in Japan.[2] As William Lee Rand explains, she did it to protect Reiki practitioners from persecution. The method had begun to gain a following in the United States around the outbreak of World War II and risked falling under the curse of anything that was Japanese.[3] Apart from this, Takata remained a controversial person in the Reiki world, especially in Japan, for ignoring some of the original rules

---

1. Lübeck et al., *The Spirit of Reiki*, 14.
2. Lübeck et al., *The Spirit of Reiki*, 24–25.
3. Lübeck et al., *The Spirit of Reiki*, 25.

and techniques while adding new ones, as well as for requiring high fees for initiation.[4]

Reiki is present today throughout the world in dozens of forms. The multitude of disciples who followed on the lineage opened by Usui have created their own schools, made changes, or added new elements to the original method; some tried to give it a more scientific look, while others emphasized a more esoteric side. Rand defines four characteristics that define the essence of any Reiki school: One cannot become a healer by reading books or by assisting at lectures but only by receiving initiation from a consecrated master; the Reiki master must belong to a lineage starting with Usui; the healing energy is not guided by one's own wisdom, but by a higher power that controls the whole healing session; and Reiki cannot have negative effects.[5]

Rather than using multiple sources to present and comment on Reiki, which would have made this chapter too long and possibly confusing, I chose to rely on three important authors: Walter Lübeck, Frank Arjava Petter, and William Lee Rand, who are leading figures in Reiki worldwide. Their book *The Spirit of Reiki: The Complete Handbook of the Reiki System* would be sufficient for a complete introduction to Reiki.

5.1 THE NATURE OF REIKI ENERGY

The Reiki healing technique is a method of directing *Ki*, the so-called "vital energy," that in Hinduism is called *prana*, and in Chinese Taoism *Chi*, which we will also encounter in acupuncture and reflexology.[6] *Rei* is the "spirit" or "hidden force" which controls the flow of *Ki* energy.[7] In Rand's view, it has a more personal ground, as he calls it "the Higher Intelligence that guides the creation and functioning of the universe," "a subtle wisdom that penetrates everything," or simply "God."[8] The spiritual teachings of Reiki on human nature combine elements from Hinduism, Buddhism, Taoism,

---

4. The fee she asked was US$ 10,000 for an initiation course over a weekend, which back in 1970 could be the price of a modest house.

5. Lübeck et al., *The Spirit of Reiki*, 22–23.

6. Walter Lübeck confirms that *Ki* is an equivalent of *prana* (Lübeck et al., *The Spirit of Reiki*, 53).

7. Lübeck et al., *The Spirit of Reiki*, 50.

8. Rand, *Reiki for a New Millennium*, 4.

Shamanism, and Gnosticism. In Lübeck's words, "a significant origin of the system is certainly the primal, shamanically oriented Chinese Taoism."[9]

Walter Lübeck explains that *Ki* energy is present in human nature in seven forms, each associated with a *chakra*. The seven forms are: *Kekki, Shioke, Mizuke, Kuki, Denki, Jiki,* and *Reiki*.[10] The first, *Kekki*, is the lowest and least structured, the raw material for the following forms. The second, *Shioke*, is a kind of anti-entropic energy, which "creates the existence of the individual," that is, individualizes *Kekki* for a personal existence. These first two forms of energy, *Kekki* and *Shioke*, are associated with the first *chakra*. The third form, *Mizuke*, relates to the second *chakra* and makes possible communication between individuals, or, in Reiki terms, the interaction between two individualized energies. The fourth, *Kuki*, generates self-consciousness, thought and direction to follow, being linked with the third *chakra*. The fifth, *Denki*, corresponds to the fourth *chakra* (the heart *chakra*). It generates moral consciousness, feelings, and provides the social component of human life. *Jiki* is the sixth form of *Ki* energy, which generates one's personality, will, aesthetics, talents, and is associated with the fifth *chakra*. Finally, Reiki is "the form of *Ki* that organizes the correct synergetic application of all the subordinate forms of the life force."[11] It is a kind of life energy that "in the material world, is closest to the divine creative force, the source of all life" and thus is called the "soul force."[12] It is connected with the sixth *chakra*, that of wisdom. The seventh *chakra* is related to what Lübeck calls the "*divine Ki*," called *Shinki*, a sort of impersonal Brahman "from which everything is created and to which everything returns after the end of its material existence."[13] In this hierarchy Reiki is the link between the individual and the ultimate reality. This is why its balancing is so important.

Unlike in the Hindu view we met in Hatha Yoga, where energy blockages must be removed so that *Kundalini* can rise from the first to the seventh *chakra*, Reiki energy enters through the fourth and the seventh *chakras* and needs to flow freely through the spiritual body so that the physical body may be healthy. If obstacles are removed at the level of all *chakras*, the free flow of *Ki* will ensure not only physical healing, but will also open the way for spiritual enlightenment. Some healers use crystals as

---

9. Lübeck et al., *The Spirit of Reiki*, 52.
10. Lübeck et al., *The Spirit of Reiki*, 52–60.
11. Lübeck et al., *The Spirit of Reiki*, 59.
12. Lübeck et al., *The Spirit of Reiki*, 59.
13. Lübeck et al., *The Spirit of Reiki*, 60.

catalysts for the inflow of energy or as absorbers of the negative energies we have accumulated.[14]

Although Usui was a Buddhist, Reiki spirituality seems to be closer to the teachings of Hinduism and of modern New Age. Lübeck states that "everyone is God, because his or her innermost core is divine."[15] The spiritual self is called "the small flame of spiritual awareness" by Petter,[16] "our divine center"[17] and "our true divine self"[18] by Lübeck, and is located in the *hara* (the second *chakra* in the Hindu representation). Illusion and ignorance keep us from knowing our nature, so we must bear the consequences of karma, which manifests as our particular condition in this life, including our health problems. Reincarnation is fully accepted in Reiki as the way we are properly rewarded for things done in previous lives. Lübeck asserts reincarnation following a Gnostic view, according to which we are angels who fell into physical bodies in order to be purified and evolve spiritually.[19]

Health issues manifest as a result of disruptions in the *Ki* energy flow. In the words of Rand, "all illness is caused by disturbances in the healthy flow of Ki within the subtle energy system."[20] As in other forms of alternative medicine, we find the Hindu picture of the four bodies which constitute human nature, among which the causal body preserves the past lives' karma. The non-physical bodies can be visualized by masters of various esoteric movements as an entity called the aura.[21] According to Rand, this

---

14. The patient lies on his back with crystals (of quartz, calcite, fluorite, etc.) placed on each *chakra*, in order to enhance Reiki treatment. There is a special Reiki form dedicated to the use of crystals, called Gemstone Reiki.

15. Lübeck, *The Complete Reiki Handbook*, 16.

16. Lübeck et al., *The Spirit of Reiki*, 91.

17. Lübeck et al., *The Spirit of Reiki*, 108.

18. Lübeck et al., *The Spirit of Reiki*, 129.

19. He says that "many angels are waiting in line to receive the opportunity for self-realization in the material world" (Lübeck et al., *The Spirit of Reiki*, 256.).

20. Lübeck et al., *The Spirit of Reiki*, 62. Rand is the founder of Karuna Reiki and of Usui Tibetan Reiki. He got to know Reiki after being a hypnotherapist involved in past-life regressions, astrologist, Tarot-card reader, and a Shaman initiated by a Hawaiian Kahuna (Lübeck et al., *The Spirit of Reiki*, 63).

21. In Rand's words, the aura is "a field of subtle energy that penetrates and extends out from the physical body" (Lübeck et al., *The Spirit of Reiki*, 87). An attempt to prove that the aura is a scientific fact led to the creation of devices that allegedly take a picture of it, such as the Kirlian AuraCam 6000. One stands in front of this "camera" with the palms resting on sensors, the picture is taken, and when it is printed it depicts the subject surrounded by a colorful cloud. This cloud is said to be the image of one's aura, while

is the place where sickness begins, "often as karma brought in from past lives or as negative *Ki*, formed by your subconscious mind in this life."[22] This negative energy affects the *chakras* and then the physical body, generating diseases.[23] Therefore the healer must first fix the energy imbalance by sending positive *Ki* energy towards the aura of the patient and thus replace his or her negative energy. Once the energy imbalance is fixed, the physical organs will heal as a result.

The karmic origin of diseases is the reason invoked for explaining why Reiki does not heal all particular health problems. If one's karma has not yet come to fruition, healing would only delay his or her spiritual evolution. In other words, if the patient owes his or her illness to "sins" committed in previous lives, the law of karma requires that they are punished by the present suffering of the patient, and thus forced healing would only postpone the necessary karmic retribution and delay one's spiritual development.

5.2 ATTEMPTED SCIENTIFIC EXPLANATIONS

As Chopra was trying to find a scientific confirmation for Ayurveda, so Rand does for Reiki. He argues that a scientific confirmation of Reiki energy is found at the level of our cells, for we know that "electric currents flow in and between all cells of the body" and that the blood vessels "allow the 'heart electricity' to flow to every part of the body."[24] Beyond this awkward paraphrasing of medical literature concerning the electrical activity of the human body, what we know is that the nervous system produces electrical activity, which can be measured by scientific investigation methods such as electroencephalography (EEG) or the electrocardiogram (EKG). The EEG records the electrical activity of the brain, while the EKG that of the heart. These are interpreted against what is considered a normal electrical activity,

---

its colors tell of his or her spiritual evolution. However, the whole story is nothing but a hoax. The electrodes record the electrical resistance of the skin, which depends on the emotional state of the person being "photographed," and according to this electric measurement, a diffuse color light overlaps the real image according to a predetermined algorithm. The colors of the "aura" change from one picture to another depending on the emotional state of the photographed person without any connection to his or her alleged spiritual bodies. For more information on this topic see: www.clarity-of-being.org/aura-photos-deception.htm.

22. Lübeck et al., *The Spirit of Reiki*, 87.
23. Lübeck et al., *The Spirit of Reiki*, 65.
24. Lübeck et al., *The Spirit of Reiki*, 71.

hence a medical doctor can draw conclusions about the health of the brain or heart.

After mentioning the normal electrical activity of our nervous system, Rand argues that the human electromagnetic field is "similar to what we call the aura" or it could be "one of the main components of the aura."[25] This conceptual leap is, however, complete fiction. The aura, Reiki energy, *Chi*, *Ki* or *prana* are concepts that do not belong to the physical world and cannot be measured by scientific means. Therefore, the idea that the "healing energy in the hands" would be generated by the "perineural system"[26] cannot have any scientific basis. If the palms of the Reiki healer were a channel for a measurable electromagnetic energy, medical science would produce a device that could emit such physical waves in a controlled and measurable way for each disease and organ. Such a device would not be guided "from a superconscious source within us,"[27] but by a medical doctor, based on a scientifically established and tested algorithm.

An attempt to scientifically prove the existence of the aura, not only by Reiki healers, but also in other forms of alternative medicine, is made by invoking the so-called Kirlian effect. In 1939 the Russian engineer Semyon Kirlian accidentally discovered that a living being or part of it (for example, a leaf or a finger) placed in a high-intensity electrical field produces an image on a photographic film in which it appears surrounded by a luminous body, as if extending from it. This has been taken as scientific evidence for the existence of the aura, *Chi* energy, the meridians of acupuncture, the etheric body, the astral body, that is, the non-physical components of human nature affirmed and healed in alternative medicine.

However, the Kirlian effect has a purely physical explanation. Any living being contains water and perspires. The electrical field charges the water vapors, and between them and the electrodes appear multiple tiny electrical discharges. These discharges produce the luminous cloud that surrounds the photographed object. In physics this electrical phenomenon is called the corona effect.

If a fresh leaf is used, the effect is strong, but as time passes, the image becomes weaker. This is not due to the loss of the etheric body following the "death" of the leaf, but to the simple fact that the leaf is losing water and no longer produces vapors that can be charged in the electrical field.

25. Lübeck et al., *The Spirit of Reiki*, 72.
26. Lübeck et al., *The Spirit of Reiki*, 73.
27. Lübeck et al., *The Spirit of Reiki*, 75.

A person sweats more or less according to his or her emotional state, so a photograph of a hand will show a stronger or weaker corona effect. If one is in a good mood, for example in the presence of a loved one, sweat is more abundant, and the Kirlian image is more prominent. The aural, etheric or astral interpretation of Kirlian photography is therefore fallacious. What is really recorded is the effect of more or less sweat, depending on the emotional state of that person, not the image of the aura or of another kind of "immaterial" body.

Therefore, Kirlian imaging does not prove that in the case of a dead body we cannot see the aura because the etheric body has "left" the physical body. A dead body no longer produces an electrical effect simply by failing to produce sweat. As a confirmation of the purely physical explanation of the Kirlian effect, under vacuum conditions no "aura" of a living organism can be recorded because there is no medium to sustain the water vapors among which the electrical discharges can occur.[28]

Another pseudo-scientific theory attempts to explain how Reiki healers can perform healings at a considerable distance. Starting with level II of Reiki, they claim that healing energy can be transmitted by using a picture of the patient or a toy that personifies the patient, which bears a striking resemblance to voodoo practice. Rand attempts to explain "scientifically" such remote healings by assuming that Reiki energy is transmitted at a distance as "scalar waves," which do "not interact with electrons as magnetic fields do, but with atomic nuclei."[29] This hypothesis is, however, sheer nonsense. Scalar waves simply do not exist for science. References to "scalar waves" can be found only in books and websites dedicated to science fiction and paranormal phenomena. As if anticipating that such a "scientific" explanation lacks credibility, Rand provides another account of how distant healing works, which speaks of the involvement of "higher beings."[30] Not having a physical body, and thus not limited by space, these beings effect healing without recourse to "magnetic fields" or "scalar waves."

Therefore the explanation of how Reiki works must be sought in the spiritual world, which is abundantly represented in this form of healing.

---

28. For more information on the Kirlian effect and its "paranormal" applications see Stenger, *Physics and Psychics*, 241–73; Watkins and Bickel, "A Study of the Kirlian Effect," 244–57.

29. Lübeck et al., *The Spirit of Reiki*, 75.

30. Lübeck et al., *The Spirit of Reiki*, 76.

5.3 THE ROLE OF SPIRITUAL BEINGS IN REIKI

One important aspect to remember is that spiritual power for healing in Reiki does not come from one's inner resources, but from the outside, and can transform a newcomer into a Reiki master very quickly. The three levels of Reiki training can each be accomplished in a short time, as quick as a weekend course per level, unlike in other forms of alternative medicine, for example acupuncture, in which training lasts for a lifetime.[31] This is why initiation is so important, and understanding what initiation means will reveal a better picture of the spiritual grounds of Reiki.

In order to become a Reiki healer one needs to be initiated in this practice by a master who belongs to the lineage of masters started by Usui. The master who conducts the initiation connects himself or herself to the Universal Source, visualizes it as a sphere of light, and then directs it to the aura of the disciple, thus transmitting him or her the power to use Reiki energy. It is a replication of the experience of Usui himself when he discovered this technique. Lübeck affirms that initiation is similar to that of other religious traditions, ranging from "Taoist initiations (Qigong and magic), transmissions of Barraka by the Sufis, Shaktipat in Hinduism, Tantric initiations, Kriya Yoga, shamanic initiations into a certain medicine power, initiations into a magical lodge in a certain degree of power of a deity."[32] As in Siddha Yoga, it can be accompanied by the manifestation of paranormal powers (*siddhis*).[33] Christine Core, the co-founder of Angelic Reiki, mentions headaches, temporary loss of memory, flu-like symptoms, crying for no reason, abnormal sweating, muscular aches and joint pain, heart arrhythmia, palpitations, sore throat, increased sensitivity, depression, etc.[34] Such manifestations must not frighten the healer, but be taken as a confirmation that he or she is following the process of unlimited spiritual growth.

Rand recounts from the experience of his own initiation, which took place in 1981: "I saw a new energy coming down through my crown *chakra* and then into my heart where it exploded out."[35] Unlike other forms of "spiritual" energy, Reiki energy is not directed by one's mind, but flows

---

31. Rand encourages potential enthusiasts that "anyone can learn it (Reiki) in a day or two and experience effective results immediately!" (Lübeck et al., *The Spirit of Reiki*, 69.).

32. Lübeck et al., *The Spirit of Reiki*, 118.

33. Lübeck et al., *The Spirit of Reiki*, 132.

34. Core, *Angelic Reiki*, 94–108.

35. Lübeck et al., *The Spirit of Reiki*, 66.

by itself, seeming "to have a mind of its own."[36] To Rand it seemed to be constituted by some "small particles of light (. . .) guided by a superior intelligence," and of a higher status than the forms of *Ki* energy he had known through previous esoteric practices.[37] It was flowing without effort, without meditation or breathing exercises, seeming to come from outside, "from a seemingly unlimited supply."[38] Rand explains that the "intention" of Reiki energy is to connect us with the "higher dimension," "to the part of the universe where all is guided by wisdom, love, and peace," to a higher experience to which it wants us to be conformed.[39]

Unlike in acupuncture or reflexology, in which the healer needs to know exactly where the intervention point is, Rand states that "Reiki doesn't have to be guided by the conscious mind of the healer, but directs itself and does not use the healer's own personal energy."[40] For this reason the Reiki healer does not follow a complicated examination procedure of the patient as in other forms of alternative medicine. Petter requires that the healer should pray, not just for the energy to flow freely and heal the patient, but to the energy itself, so that it may guide his or her hands to the sick organ. He instructs: "Ask the Reiki power to flow through you" and "to guide your hands to where the energy is needed."[41] As a result of such prayers, the energy will respond by tactile, auditory or visual sensations or even with voices or visions.[42] Likewise, Lübeck urges the healer to ask "permission to be a channel for Reiki "[43] and, at the end of the healing session, to be thankful to have been "allowed to be a Reiki energy channel."[44] This astonishing simplicity of Reiki healing raises questions about what or who might be the higher intellect which controls Reiki energy, since energy itself cannot have a mind or will to guide the hands of the healer.

We can suspect that this energy is not just an *it*, but has a personal nature and source. In other words, Reiki energy does not act autonomously as claimed, but is directed by mysterious spiritual beings. Lübeck affirms

36. Lübeck et al., *The Spirit of Reiki*, 66.
37. Lübeck et al., *The Spirit of Reiki*, 66–67.
38. Lübeck et al., *The Spirit of Reiki*, 66–67.
39. Lübeck et al., *The Spirit of Reiki*, 70.
40. Lübeck et al., *The Spirit of Reiki*, 74.
41. Usui and Petter, *The Original Reiki Handbook*, 17.
42. Lübeck et al., *The Spirit of Reiki*, 150–51.
43. Lübeck et al., *The Spirit of Reiki*, 208.
44. Lübeck et al., *The Spirit of Reiki*, 216.

that Reiki has a patron deity called Dainichi Nyorei,[45] which is the Japanese name of Buddha Vairocana, one of the five Dhyani Buddhas of Tibetan Buddhism.[46] Among many such spiritual beings invoked in Reiki we find the "archangels" Michael and Gabriel, Egyptian gods, or the Tibetan goddess Kuan Yin. Rand demands that the healing session be prepared by calling in "the ancestors and the ascended masters and Reiki guides asking them to bless you and your client and to help you with your healing treatment."[47] This is not just an imaginary exercise, since he argues that "many (healers) have reported that they felt additional hands on them and the presence of someone else in the room during a Reiki treatment."[48]

The religious character of Reiki thus becomes more and more obvious, despite insistence that it is not a religion, but a "spiritual path" born out of "a religious experience" of its founder, Usui.[49] As Lübeck himself affirms, it is not just a healing technique, but a "mystic path to the light," which "only opens up to those who are truly willing to look into the clear mirror of the divine self."[50] This "mystic path" leads us to a finality similar to that of Yoga, that is, to uniting our "divine self" with "the Great Divine Light."[51] Physical healing is only a secondary goal, while the ultimate goal is spiritual enlightenment. For this reason, Lübeck emphasizes that in the case of an incurable disease "the challenge is to delay death until the sick person becomes aware of his own divine spark."[52]

The fact that we are dealing with a new religious movement, instead of just a new form of healing, is also revealed by the use of auditory and visual tools similar to those of Hinduism. Lübeck recommends the recitation of the initiation mantra over "100,000 times during favorable astrological periods" and admits that this recitation is "connected with a sequence of visualizations of mantras and invocations of the respective deities in states of deep meditation."[53] In a similar way to Transcendental Meditation, it is

---

45. Lübeck et al., *The Spirit of Reiki*, 121.

46. In the *Tibetan Book of the Dead*, the Buddha Vairocana is the first being who offers himself to guide the deceased to the light of nirvana.

47. Rand, *Reiki for a New Millennium*, 29.

48. Rand, *Reiki for a New Millennium*, 32.

49. Lübeck et al., *The Spirit of Reiki*, 93.

50. Lübeck et al., 245–46.

51. Lübeck et al., 249.

52. Lübeck, *The Complete Reiki Handbook*, 28.

53. Lübeck et al., *The Spirit of Reiki*, 118.

claimed that the correct use of mantras will "evoke their associated spirits to the person using Reiki."[54]

The visual tools used in Reiki are called symbols. They are simple drawings that have the role of *yantras* in Hinduism or *mandalas* in Tibetan Buddhism.[55] There are specific symbols to invoke various spirits and deities, such as the Buddhist female deity Kuan Yin (Tara, in Tibet), the Egyptian god Horus, or Avalokiteshvara,[56] the supreme Tibetan bodhisattva. In using a certain symbol, although it is explicitly intended to contact spirits, Lübeck says that to transfer "any hostile forces – destructive in the spiritual sense – is impossible."[57] However, as Christians, we should remember the words of the apostle Paul, who warns us that "even Satan masquerades as an angel of light," and "his ministers also masquerade as ministers of righteousness" (2 Cor 11,14–15) in order to delude us. This explanation looks highly probable, especially as we look to the whole of Reiki doctrines and the spiritual direction in which they lead us.[58]

5.4 REIKI AND CHRISTIANITY

Reiki is a form of New Age spirituality in which all religions are valid paths to the same ultimate reality. Rand affirms that it can be called "God, the Supreme Being, The Universe, The Universal Mind, All That Is, Jehovah, Krishna, Buddha, The Great Spirit, etc." [59] All spiritual paths are valid, and one has to find the one that best fits himself or herself.[60] However, such syncretistic views on ultimate reality are false, both for Buddhists and for

---

54. Lübeck et al., *The Spirit of Reiki*, 124.

55. The *yantras* are diagrams used in Yoga and Tantra to enhance concentration, while *mandalas* are more elaborate drawings used in Tibetan Buddhism for the same purpose.

56. Lübeck et al., *The Spirit of Reiki*, 129.

57. Lübeck et al., *The Spirit of Reiki*, 126.

58. Another form of alternative medicine in which spirits are involved is shamanic medicine. The shaman, also called the medicine man, is one who enters a trance state (by the use of hallucinogenic drugs, ritual dance, chanting and drumming) and travels to the world of spirits to fetch the necessary information for the cure of his patient. Like Reiki, it is a form of contacting a world of spirits which are not God's angels, for the Bible and Church teaching explicitly forbid this practice (see Deut 18,9–14 and the *Catechism of the Catholic Church* 2116–17).

59. Lübeck et al., *The Spirit of Reiki*, 68.

60. Lübeck et al., *The Spirit of Reiki*, 93.

Christians. On the one hand, Buddhism, to which Usui belonged, does not admit the existence of a permanent ultimate reality, of a personal or an impersonal nature, not even the Brahman of Hinduism. Buddhism admits only an everlasting truth, that of impermanence (*anitya*), meaning there is *no* ultimate reality, and that everything is the result of change.[61]

On the other hand, in Christianity, the Holy Trinity is not an equivalent of all the above mentioned deities, and Jesus is not just one among many spiritual masters. He is not just a revealer of one of many paths, the teacher of one of many truths, and one of many examples of how to live, but *the* way, *the* truth and *the* life (John 14,6). Therefore when we examine the relationship between Reiki spirituality and Christian teachings, it is obvious that Reiki is an invitation to experience a whole different spiritual path. Any attempt to reconcile Reiki with Christianity must consider the following theological issues:

- God is the Holy Trinity, three consubstantial Persons, not an impersonal energy called the Great Divine Light, Universal Light, Universal Source, universal vital force, cosmic energy, or anything else.

- Jesus is not *one of many* spiritual masters of mankind, but the only Savior and Lord, the Son of God, of one substance with the Father.

- The Holy Spirit is not a healing energy that we can guide through a technique, but a Person of the Holy Trinity.

- Angels are not servants of initiated people, but of God, and they cannot work contrary to God's will and revelation, unless they are fallen angels, called demons.

- Human beings do not have a divine inner nature, or a core of the same nature as that of God. Like everything else in God's creation, we are preserved in existence by his grace.

- The significance of sin and the need for repentance for sins are completely ignored in Reiki because there is no supreme God, against whom one may sin.

- Divine healing is received by God's grace and leads to the strengthening of one's faith and to a virtuous life. It is not the result of energy adjustment with a universal vital force and cannot lead to appropriating New Age beliefs.

---

61. You can find a brief introduction to Buddhism in chapter 7, section 5.

Despite these fundamental issues, Reiki masters still claim that Christians can and should use this form of therapy. *Reiki for Christians*, although a contradiction in terms, is the name of a website that encourages Christians to use Reiki. It affirms that:

> Scripture clearly indicates that healing is something appropriate for Christians to be involved with. Christians who have a solid foundation in their faith know that God will always protect and guide them. Those Christians who practice Reiki do so within the guidance and protection of God secure in the belief that they have been guided to follow Jesus' example to be a healer.[62]

As we can see, Reiki is presented as an ancient form of healing practiced by Jesus himself. Rand proposes two ways of explaining how Reiki and Christianity find their common ground in Jesus: Either he was himself initiated in Reiki in the Far East and then used it back home in Palestine,[63] or his disciples taught it in the Far East and it became incorporated into Tibetan Buddhism. Eventually it was lost for centuries and rediscovered by Usui.[64] However, to see Jesus as a palm healer is a great misrepresentation of both his identity and his healing power. Jesus did not heal primarily by laying his hands on sick people, but by his words. The use of hands was just the visible sign of the spoken word, and this sign could be lacking. On a careful examination of Jesus' healings in the Gospels, we see that the cases in which he verbally proclaimed one's healing are more numerous than those in which he used his hands.[65] His healing of people by spoken words follows the way God the Father brought the world into existence by his word. As such, his healings point to his divine nature, not to a skill in using a universal energy. If he had used an "ancient" Reiki technique, Jesus would have been a mere channel for the flow of universal energy, not the very Source, Light of Light, very God of very God, as we affirm in the Creed. In a document called "Guidelines for Evaluating Reiki as an Alternative Therapy," issued by the US Conference of Catholic Bishops, we are warned against such deception:

> Some people have attempted to identify Reiki with the divine healing known to Christians. They are mistaken. (. . .) the fact remains

---

62. *Reiki for Christians*, online.
63. Rand, *Reiki for a New Millennium*, 88.
64. Rand, *Reiki for a New Millennium*, 91.
65. Of the 24 healings that I could count in the gospels (including exorcisms), in 11 cases Jesus used his hands, while in another 13 he did not.

that for Christians the access to divine healing is by prayer to Christ as Lord and Savior, while the essence of Reiki is not a prayer but a technique that is passed down from the "Reiki Master" to the pupil, a technique that once mastered will reliably produce the anticipated results.[66]

Another potentially convincing argument, which concerns mostly Catholic and Eastern Orthodox Christians, is seen in the laying on of hands by a bishop when bestowing the sacrament of priesthood. As the argument goes, since the word "ordination" means "laying hands" (*cheirotonia*, in Greek), in Reiki we can see it applied in both initiation and healing. But does this mean that the same thing happens in Reiki? It obviously does not, for in ordination what is transmitted is not an energy, but an authority, by which the bishop delegates to the newly ordained priest the power of bestowing the sacraments. In the act of ordination, the laying on of hands is the outward sign that grace flows from the bishop to the new priest following a lineage that started with the apostles of Jesus. They were delegated by Christ himself to represent him in the world and, in their turn, delegated other bishops as Christianity spread throughout the world. In other words, the laying on of hands in ordination is the visible sign that accompanies the delegation of this authority on the line of apostolic succession, not a flow of energy from one person to another. This is why the Catholic Catechism says that "the priest, by virtue of the sacrament of Holy Orders, acts *in persona Christi Capitis*."[67] It means that the priest acts in place of Christ, the one from whom priestly authority originates.

Another aspect of Reiki that should raise serious concerns to Christians is the teaching on sin. In the Bible sin is viewed as a moral barrier that makes it impossible to live in a covenant of grace with God. The prophet Isaiah says: "Your iniquities have separated you from your God; your sins have hidden his face from you, so that he will not hear" (Isa 59,2). The incarnation of Christ, his teachings, his death on the cross, and his resurrection are essential elements on which Christianity is founded, and by which he brought our delivery from sin. In Reiki spirituality, however, the problem of sin is seen very differently. Sin is not a moral barrier between us and God, but an illusion.[68] Instead of sin, in the Christian sense, in Reiki

---

66. United States Conference of Catholic Bishops, *Guidelines for Evaluating Reiki*, paragraph 8.

67. CCC 1548.

68. Lübeck, *The Complete Reiki Handbook*, 15.

Reiki

they speak of ignorance, in the Hindu sense. For instance, in dealing with anger, Lübeck affirms that it should be seen as a "powerful energy" that has been sent to us by the "Higher Self."[69] Instead of repentance, we need to imagine "how this power can be meaningfully translated into actions," for instance by the use of "meditation on a regular basis, and intensive oracle work."[70]

The most striking element in Reiki is without doubt the help provided by "divinities," "angels," or "spiritual beings," that is, the spirits invoked for initiation and healing. In the first level of Reiki they are barely mentioned, but in the master level they get primary attention. According to Christian teaching, angels are indeed immaterial beings, but contrary to Reiki teaching, they are not our servants, but God's messengers. They are not like the genie that comes out of Aladdin's lamp and fulfills any desire.

Therefore, the "spiritual beings" of Reiki, who present themselves with a different mission and uphold teachings contrary to basic Christian teachings, must be another kind of angels. They are fallen angels, called demons, and their goal is to deceive us. The apostle Peter warns us: "Discipline yourselves, keep alert. Like a roaring lion your adversary the devil prowls around, looking for someone to devour" (1 Pet 5,8). The apostle John, in his turn, wrote to his disciples: "Beloved, do not believe every spirit, but test the spirits to see whether they are from God; for many false prophets have gone out into the world" (1 John 4,1). Knowing what the angels of Reiki teach, we have serious reason to doubt that they are God's angels. A true angel does not distort Christian teachings, does not teach karma and reincarnation, that we have a divine nature, but confirms what Christians have always taught and especially the need for repentance for sins. Therefore the "angels" of Reiki must be demons.

Since Reiki spirituality systematically contradicts fundamental Christian teachings, do we still need to ponder whether it can be used by a Christian, as a healer or as a patient? Lübeck reassures his readers that "members of any faith can learn Reiki without leaving their own spiritual tradition."[71] This may be true for the followers of esoteric and syncretistic religious movements, which already have a common ground with Reiki, but not for Christians. Contrary to Lübeck's words, Reiki cannot offer "a personal encounter with the divine – independent of any church, sect or

---

69. Lübeck et al., *The Spirit of Reiki*, 250.
70. Lübeck et al., *The Spirit of Reiki*, 250–51.
71. Lübeck et al., *The Spirit of Reiki*, 135.

holy writing,"[72] or, according to Rand, "a more immediate experience of the divine."[73] More than being merely incompatible with Christian faith, the use of Reiki is synonymous with breaking the first commandment. Although Rand claims that Reiki "cannot do harm and always works for the positive benefit of the client,"[74] the danger is real, and is called apostasy.

5.5 ADDENDUM. THERAPEUTIC TOUCH AND MACROBIOTICS

Another form of palm-healing known in the Western world is Therapeutic Touch (TT). Its founders, Dolores Krieger and Dora Kunz (former president of the Theosophical Society), are heavily influenced by New Age teachings. TT works on the assumption that "a human being is an open energy system" and therefore "the transfer of energy between people is a natural, continuous event."[75] The centers that distribute energy to the body are the seven *chakras*. Krieger calls them "transformers of energy" and "centers of different levels of consciousness."[76] Illness is considered "an imbalance in an individual's energy field,"[77] and healing is produced through the transfer of energy from healer to patient through the secondary *chakras* located in the palms.[78]

The healing session takes 10–20 minutes and consists of several stages: First, both the healer and the patient engage in a short meditation, called "centering," in order to become sensitive to the flow of energy. Then follows the assessment of the patient's health, by scanning his or her aura with the palms held a few inches above the skin, from head to feet, frontal and dorsal. During this procedure the healer has diverse sensations in the palms, such as heat, cold, heaviness, or tingling, which signal health problems.

---

72. Lübeck et al., *The Spirit of Reiki*, 135.

73. Lübeck et al., *The Spirit of Reiki*, 269. Therefore, Lübeck's insistence that in the case of an incurable disease "the challenge is to delay death until the sick person becomes aware of his own divine spark" (Lübeck, *The Complete Reiki Handbook*, 28), would for a Christian translate as a requirement to delay death until the sick person gives away his or her saving faith.

74. Lübeck et al., *The Spirit of Reiki*, 69.

75. Krieger, *Personal Practice*, 12.

76. Krieger, *Personal Practice*, 23.

77. Krieger, *Personal Practice*, 12.

78. Krieger, *Personal Practice*, 23.

The actual healing consists of "unruffling," that is, decongesting the energy field of the patient, and transferring energy to the patient. At this stage the healer feels a reversal of the sensations had during diagnosis (cool places are warmed up, hot points are cooled down). In the end the healer assesses the session and closes the procedure.

Unlike in Reiki, in TT there is no initiation ritual involved. One learns the skills by assisting a healer and by developing his or her own abilities. The healer actively directs the flow of energy, and is not a mere channel for it, as in Reiki. This technique does not claim to heal critical conditions, but is limited to bringing relaxation, reducing pain and accelerating the body's natural healing capacity. A Christian should realize that, although there are no "angelic" beings invoked in TT, it is heavily influenced by esoteric teachings and that it reduces human nature to an "energy system."

Macrobiotics is another form of palm-healing, founded by the Japanese George Ohsawa (born Nyoichi Sakurazawa) (1893–1966). In the Western world it was promoted by Michio Kushi (1926–2014), Ohsawa's disciple and author of many best-selling books. Although macrobiotics is known mostly by its miraculous diet for weight loss, it is a form of alternative medicine that goes into deep esoteric teachings which combine Hindu pantheism and Taoism.

Kushi mentions "sixteen different methods of diagnosis, all of which are derived from the understanding of the order of the universe, or natural law."[79] The first is astrology, or "Heavenly Phenomena," which "is based on the influence of the different types of celestial motion that affect human life."[80] Another one is "Spiritual Diagnosis," which "involves being able to perceive the influences exerted by people who have died."[81] According to Kushi, the spirits of persons we had a special relationship with remain attached to us as ghosts and influence our daily lives. Other spirits that affect us are "wandering spirits," which belong to persons who were mistreated by us or by our ancestors and need to be pacified.[82] Astrology and ghosts are just two of the factors that influence our physical and mental health.

Some diagnostic methods are taken from traditional Chinese medicine. These include studying the relationships between organs that reflect

---

79. Kushi, *Natural Healing*, 49.
80. Kushi, *Natural Healing*, 49.
81. Kushi, *Natural Healing*, 55.
82. Kushi, *Natural Healing*, 56.

the relationships between the five elements,[83] taking the pulses, and examining the face, tongue, and odors. Almost like a special form of reflexology, the tip of the nose corresponds to the heart, the place between eyebrows corresponds to the liver, the middle point of the cheeks corresponds to the lungs, etc.[84]

Another assessing method is similar to TT's scanning the energy field of a patient with the palms, with special emphasis on the *chakras*.[85] The *chakras* are energy centers which collect and distribute Ki energy to the body, each *chakra* to its associated group of organs and mental abilities. Macrobiotics combines the Hindu *chakra* representation of human nature with the Chinese meridian theory as we know it from acupuncture, claiming that the meridians branch out of the *sushumna* channel to all regions of the body "nourishing us with vital force."[86]

Both the healer and the patient need to prepare for treatment by engaging in meditation. The aura of the patient is diagnosed by a palm-scan and then purified of its negative energies by the inflow of positive energy through the hands of the healer. Then follows a more focused energy treatment of the affected organs. An associated practice is the recitation of mantras, especially of the Hindu mantra *AUM*, in order to increase effectiveness in dispersing negative energies. Instead of its Hindu purpose, that of leading one to oneness with ultimate reality, in macrobiotics the chanting of the *AUM* mantra is said to have healing effects. Its three letters stimulate individual *chakras* as follows:

> "Ah" stimulates the abdominal *chakra* and the digestive system as a whole, along with the lungs and respiratory system. "Uu" is a more balanced sound, and activates the heart region and circulatory system. "Mm" energizes the midbrain in particular and the nervous system in general.[87]

Unlike Reiki, macrobiotics does not explicitly invoke "angels" or deities for help. However, its esoteric view of human nature, which combines elements of Hinduism and Taoism, such as *yin-yang*, *chakras*, universal energy, etc., can be seductive for Christians. In a way that combines Hindu pantheism with Taoism, Kushi affirms: "Our life in this space and time is a

---

83. Kushi, *Natural Healing*, 75–78.
84. Kushi wrote a whole book on this topic: *Your Face Never Lies*.
85. Kushi, *Macrobiotics and Oriental Medicine*, 183.
86. Kushi, *Macrobiotic Palm Healing*, 102.
87. Kushi and Jannetta, *Macrobiotics an Oriental Medicine*, 169.

faint wave which is governed by the order of the universe, *yin* and *yang*."[88] He boldly affirms that macrobiotics is "creating a new human species; one which lives in cooperation with the forces of nature."[89] What one should take as ultimate reality is an infinite universe ruled by seven universal principles, of which the first says that "everything is a differentiation of one Infinity."[90] Since ultimate reality is an impersonal "Infinity," our destiny is "to return to Infinity again after we live as one of the human beings of this earth."[91] This is consistent with the first principle of the "macrobiotic way": "Have Unconditioned Faith in the Order of the Universe."[92]

But this is not what Christianity teaches. Ultimate Reality is God. He revealed himself as the Holy Trinity, and our unconditional faith is in him, as a Person, not in an impersonal universal order.

---

88. Kushi, *The Book of Macrobiotics*, 95.
89. Kushi, *Macrobiotics and Oriental Medicine*, 259–60.
90. Kushi, *The Book of Macrobiotics*, 7.
91. Kushi, *The Book of Macrobiotics*, 95.
92. Kushi, *The Book of Macrobiotics*, 95.

6

Acupuncture and the Principles of Traditional Chinese Medicine

ACUPUNCTURE IS A FORM of traditional Chinese medicine with deep spiritual roots in Taoism. In order to avoid "westernized" or "modernized" views of acupuncture which greatly distort it, we need to understand a few guiding principles of this ancient Chinese religion.

6.1 A BRIEF INTRODUCTION TO TAOISM

In a similar way to pantheistic Hinduism, in Taoism we meet an impersonal ultimate reality called Tao. But unlike Brahman, which is a static essence out of which everything has been manifested and in which everything returns, Tao has a more dynamic nature, resembling a force which flows continuously through all forms of life. Rather than a static essence, it is rather the source of permanent transformation, a kind of vital principle that sustains the whole universe through its flow. In the words of Eliade, "Tao is the principle of order, immanent in all the realms of the real," "a primordial totality, living and creative but formless and nameless."[1] The true significance of Tao remains hidden, and the more precisely we try to define it the more we misunderstand its essence. This is stated by the very first words of the *Tao Te Ching*, the treatise left to us by Lao Tzu (or Lao Zi), the founder of this religion, in the sixth century BC: "Even the finest teaching

---

1. Eliade, *A History of Religious Ideas*, II, 20–21.

is not the Tao itself. Even the finest name is insufficient to define it. Without words, the Tao can be experienced, and without a name, it can be known."[2]

Unlike Hinduism, Taoism does not affirm an antithesis between the physical body and an inner divine self. We do not find such a duality in Taoism, nor a drive to release a "self" from the prison of the body. What one must find by introspection is not an entity, but a mechanism that governs our nature. In the *Tao Te Ching* we read:

> The Tao may be known and observed without the need of travel; the way of the heavens might be well seen without looking through a window. The further one travels, the less one knows. So, without looking, the sage sees all, and by working without self-advancing thought, he discovers the wholeness of the Tao.[3]

In other words, the whole universe is represented in one's own nature, so from knowing ourselves we can know the whole universe, and from observing nature we can know ourselves, for we are a little replica of the universe. Ioan Couliano, a disciple of Eliade, explains that, according to the Taoist view,

> Human beings were the image of the universe. They were enlivened by a primordial breath divided into *yin* and *yang*, female and male, earth and heaven. The phenomenon of life was based on this energy hidden in its manifestations. If the energy was preserved and increased, then the human being was able to attain immortality.[4]

As Couliano point out, the Tao manifests itself as two opposing and complementary forces: *yin*, the negative, and *yang*, the positive. They are present everywhere in nature, as the alternation of winter and summer, 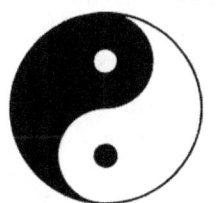 night and day, cold and heat, negative and positive, etc. The whole world seems to be represented in such opposite pairs that define each other. When one of the two forces reaches the climax of its development, the other starts to replace it. In the classical representation we are familiar with, *yin* and *yang* are represented as two tadpole-shaped halves of a circle, facing opposite directions. The boundary between them, in the form of an inverted S-shaped line, suggests their

---

2. *Tao Te Ching*, chapter 1.
3. *Tao Te Ching*, chapter 47.
4. Eliade and Couliano, *Eliade Guide to World Religions*, 238.

complementarity, and the dot of the opposite color in each half reminds us of the potential of one force to turn into its opposite. The *yin/yang* polarity exists in every aspect of the world and of human life, and therefore the ideal of Taoist spirituality is to understand this perpetual transformation and to live in harmony with it.

Unlike Hinduism, Taoism requires not the liberation of an inner self, but perfecting the body and attaining immortality. The defeat of ignorance is accomplished by living in harmony with the Tao, by finding the proper balance of its polar forces inside oneself. This is the essence of the *wu wei* doctrine, which means "acting through non-action," or in other words, cultivating a state of mind in which actions follow the flow of nature. The actual techniques of attainment of perfection, which are a kind of Taoist Yoga, are known in the Western world as Tai Chi and Qigong.

6.2 TAI CHI AND QIGONG

You have probably seen in public spaces groups of practitioners moving slowly and gracefully in unison as though they were performing a ritual dance in slow motion. Most likely they were practitioners of a Taoist tradition called Tai Chi, one of the two major forms in which we meet Taoism in the Western world. The other is Qigong.[5] Although both traditions follow the basic Taoist tenets mentioned above, there are significant differences between Tai Chi and Qigong.

Qigong (Chi Kung, or Chi Gung) means cultivating the energy of life (*Chi*). It is an ancient Chinese discipline that existed long before Lao Tzu and developed into hundreds of styles. The movements may differ significantly between styles. Most are graceful, rhythmic and repetitive, while others look more like shaking, jumping, screaming, and flapping hands along the body as if mimicking the flying of a bird. The movements are repeated several times in the same way, in correlation with breath control. Some are fast and alternate with complete rest; others are strange and spontaneous, occasionally accompanied by strong shouts. These movements and other

---

5. There exists a form of "Chinese Yoga," called *Daoyin*, in which physical exercises are used in order to guide the flow of *Chi*. In a similar way to Hindu Yoga, these exercises have a deeper purpose, not just that of keeping one healthy. As Camilo Sanchez argues, "While the term yoga is of Indian origin, it can be rightly used to describe the Daoist meridian exercises as they emphasize the integration of the body, vital energy, and mind, as well as cultivating a higher level of awareness" (Sanchez, *Daoist Meridian Yoga*, 11).

manifestations in Qigong practice are ways of conducting *Chi* energy, according to the goals of each style.

There are five main branches of Qigong, defined by their religious orientation: Confucian, Buddhist, Taoist, one related to Chinese medicine, and one related to martial arts. Each is adapted to the requirements of the associated religious beliefs. Thus Buddhist Qigong has different objectives from those of Taoist Qigong. The Qigong of martial arts aims to store *Chi* energy in the form of power, through physical exercise, controlled breathing and meditation. According to one of its masters, its aim is "to increase the power and efficiency of the muscles," and the knowledge of energy flow is used "to attack specific areas, such as vital acupuncture cavities, to disturb the enemy's *Chi* flow and create imbalances or even death."[6] Medical Qigong is particularly concerned with the intake of *Chi* energy and its harmonious distribution throughout the body. Both the Qigong for martial arts and the medical Qigong hold that we have a reservoir of *Chi* energy (called *dantien*)[7] which is filled during practice and then used as a source of power, or healing.

Tai chi (TaiJi or T'ai Chi Ch'uan)[8] originated as a form of Chinese martial art, but is practiced in the Western world mostly as a form of physical exercise for health. "Tai" means "supreme," while "ji" translates as "ultimate" or "limit," hence it could be translated literally as the "supreme limit." "Chuan" means "boxing," and thus the longer name is used mainly to refer to the martial art. Whether practiced as martial art or for health, Tai Chi practice aims to achieve the goal of Taoist spirituality, that of conforming to the ultimate harmony of the universe.[9] In Tai Chi the movements are more complex than in Qigong; they are not repetitive, but rather flow from one to the next. Although it is claimed to bring peace of mind and bodily health, good digestion and blood circulation, inner calm and long life, Tai Chi cannot be considered just a form of physical exercise or a kind of serene dance, not even in the initiation stage. The same caution mentioned in assessing the Yoga practice applies here as well. Just as Yoga does not mean mere physical exercise (*asanas*) and attaining mobility, but bringing the

---

6. Jwing-Ming, *The Essence of Tai Chi*, 14–15.

7. Its location corresponds to the second *chakra* of Hindu Hatha Yoga and Tantra.

8. The "Chi" in its name does not point to the vital force known as *Chi*.

9. A master of Tai Chi affirms: "Everything, even unfilled space, derives its existence from the balanced interaction of these two contrasting forces. Since the powers of Yin and Yang are the origin of everything, they are the ultimate nature of every object in this universe" (Liao, *T'ai Chi Classics*, 17).

body under control to make meditation possible, Tai Chi should rather be taken as a kind of Taoist Yoga, a spiritual discipline that uses breathing and meditation exercises in order that the practitioner may conform himself or herself to the flow of universal *Chi* energy.

Therefore both Tai Chi and Qigong represent more than Chinese gymnastics or a special kind of exercise for health. If they are not integrated into a Taoist spiritual discipline, the physical exercises do not achieve what they are meant for.

6.3 HUMAN ANATOMY AND PHYSIOLOGY IN ACUPUNCTURE

The oldest known treatise of traditional Chinese medicine is considered to be the *Huangdi Neijing* (*The Yellow Emperor's Classic of Medicine*), said to have been composed by the Chinese emperor Huangdi, about five millennia ago.[10] The treatise is a dialogue between Huangdi and his principal doctor, Qi Bo, in which they discuss health, disease, and proper treatment. It starts with the emperor's question:

> I've heard that in the days of old everyone lived one hundred years without showing the usual signs of aging. In our time, however, people age prematurely, living only fifty years. Is this due to a change in the environment, or is it because people have lost the correct way of life?[11]

The central idea of the treatise is that one who seeks health must live in harmony with the Tao. When *yin* and *yang* get out of balance, the physical body becomes ill. Therefore Qi Bo responds:

> In the past, people practiced the Tao, the Way of Life. They understood the principle of balance, of *yin* and *yang*, as represented by the transformation of the energies of the universe.[12]

---

10. This is the conservative view, see Kretsinger, *History and Philosophy of Biology*, 159. However, modern authors claim that Huangdi is a semi-mythical figure, and indicate a much later date for this book, not earlier than the third century BC (see: http://www.newworldencyclopedia.org/entry/Huangdi_Neijing#Date_of_composition).
11. *The Yellow Emperor's Classic of Medicine*, 1.
12. *The Yellow Emperor's Classic of Medicine*, 1.

Acupuncture and the Principles of Traditional Chinese Medicine

The essence of traditional Chinese medicine is summarized as mastering the proper *yin/yang* balance inside human nature. The emperor concludes:

> The law of *yin* and *yang* is the natural order of the universe, the foundation of all things, mother of all changes, the root of life and death. In healing, one must grasp the root of the disharmony, which is always subject to the law of *yin* and *yang*.[13]

One of the most important pioneers of acupuncture in the Western world is the French acupuncturist Georges Soulié de Morant (1878–1955), who, for his merits in promoting acupuncture, received the highest Chinese civilian award, the Coral Globe, an unprecedented achievement for a Westerner. Therefore I consider his writings of first importance in describing and assessing acupuncture, especially his book *Chinese Acupuncture*. By following Morant I intend to avoid attempts to secularize acupuncture and ignore its spiritual foundations to make it more acceptable to Westerners.

In quite a similar way to the flow of *prana* according to the Hindu view on human nature, in traditional Chinese medicine the physical body is kept alive by the flow of a vital energy called *Chi*. Manuals of acupuncture state that it flows through twelve principal channels, called meridians (*jingmai*). When the flow of *Chi* energy is affected somewhere along a meridian, the balance of *yin/yang* forces is disrupted, and as a result, a physical ailment will occur.

Ten principal meridians correspond to the main organs of the body. There are five *yin* organs, corresponding to the heart, lung,[14] liver, spleen, and kidneys, and five *yang* organs, corresponding to the small intestine, large intestine, gallbladder, stomach, and urinary bladder. Another two meridians are the one associated with the pericardium, which stands for sexuality, and the triple burner, responsible for converting food into energy. According to Morant there are two other energy channels, called median lines, which follow the anterior and posterior part of the body: the conception vessel (*ren mai*) and the governor vessel (*du mai*).[15] In addition to these Morant mentions fifteen secondary vessels that connect the twelve principal meridians.[16] He makes it clear that these energy channels do not

---

13. *The Yellow Emperor's Classic of Medicine*, 17.
14. Traditional Chinese medicine considers the "lung" a singular organ.
15. Morant, *Chinese Acupuncture*, 39.
16. Morant, *Chinese Acupuncture*, 42.

correspond to blood vessels or nerves, so it is pointless to search for their physical correspondents in classical anatomy.[17]

As we can see, the brain is not among the principal organs, nor is mental life associated with it. All aspects of mental life which could correspond to the Christian view of the soul are bound to the five *yin* organs, as the five spirits (*shen, hun, po, yi* and *zhi*). They are not components of an immaterial soul, but forms of *Chi* energy stored in the five principal *yin* organs (heart, liver, lung, spleen, and kidney).

Since there are also Confucian and Neo-Confucian influences in traditional Chinese medicine on how the five spirits work, as well as different views among Chinese scholars on this issue, I will rely on Morant's description as authoritative in order to draw a reliable picture of traditional acupuncture. His analysis states that the heart is the home of the *shen*, the master of the spirits, which is responsible for "intelligence, or reason guided by principles and morals and not by instincts or needs."[18] The *shen* seems to be the closest correspondent to what Westerners call the *mind*, since it is "the psychic director of conscience and understanding, reason, judgment, common sense, the critical capacity and consciousness; the true intelligence that understands without having learned through simple comparisons."[19] The liver stores the *hun*, which is an ethereal component that drives one's will towards higher, spiritual things, while the *po* (stored in the lung) is a corporeal component that fuels the interest for physical needs, food, sex, and possessions. Intent (*yi*) and will (*zhi*) are the last of the five spirits. The first is bound to the spleen, and the second to the kidneys. The five organs and their spirits are linked to a complex network of relationships, which includes the fundamental elements of Chinese cosmology, planets, and cardinal points, but to go into such detail would far exceed the limits of this book.[20]

---

17. Morant, *Chinese Acupuncture*, 26.
18. Morant, *Chinese Acupuncture*, 87.
19. Morant, *Chinese Acupuncture*, 616.
20. These five items are grouped as following:
East–Wood–Jupiter–Liver–*Hun*;
South–Fire–Mars–Heart–*Shen*;
West–Metal–Venus–Lungs–*Po*;
North–Water–Mercury–Kidneys–*Zhi*;
Center–Earth–Saturn–Spleen–*Yi*.

6.4 DIAGNOSIS AND TREATMENT IN ACUPUNCTURE

As we would expect, diagnosis in acupuncture follows a very different pattern from that of Western medicine. The health of organs, or more precisely of the flow of *Chi* energy through the meridians corresponding to physical organs, is assessed by examining the pulses, the body odors, the eyes, tongue, and skin, and follows an elaborate interview with the patient.

In a similar way to Ayurveda, examining the pulse has nothing to do with the physical heart rate. Instead of one's *pulse*, in acupuncture we speak of *pulses*, in the plural, because there are twelve different pulses, one for each of the twelve principal meridians. Quite similarly to Ayurveda, the pulses are taken on the radial artery, close to the left and right wrist. Three kinds of pulses are taken with three different fingers, the index, the middle, and the ring finger, at two different depths (superficial and deep), so a total of six pulses are taken with each of the examiner's hands.[21] It takes a great deal of sensitivity to perceive the differences between them, and thus practitioners need many years of training. A correct diagnosis is reached by examining pulse intensity, its firmness, the rate during one breath, and other very subtle qualities. In addition to indications from pulses, the eyes provide indications of the health of the liver, the ears inform of the health of the kidneys, the lips show the condition of the spleen, the lungs are assessed by examining the nose, while the tongue indicates the health of the heart. Claus Schnorrenberger, founder and director of the German Research Institute of Chinese Medicine (GRICMED), affirms that specialists can get additional information about the state of the principal organs by carefully observing the different parts of the eye. For example, the pupils correspond to the kidneys, the iris to the liver, the sclera (the white of the eye) to the lung, the capillaries of the sclera correspond to the heart, and the eyelids to the spleen.[22]

The physical place where the acupuncturist intervenes for restoring the *Chi* energy balance in the meridians is the acupuncture point. There are hundreds of such points; Morant mentions 618 on the 12 main meridians, plus 147 on the secondary ones, making a total of 765 points.[23] For each disease, or rather *yin/yang* imbalance, in a certain number of such points

---

21. Of the twelve pulses taken, the locations of six correspond to those of Ayurveda (heart, small intestine, kidneys, bladder, lung, and large intestine).

22. Schnorrenberger, *Chen-Chiu*, 154.

23. Morant, *Chinese Acupuncture*, 19. Other acupuncturists follow other charts, with different numbers of such points.

needles are inserted, of a certain type, at a certain depth and angle, and for a certain time. They can be rotated or heated during the treatment in a certain way.

A practice associated with acupuncture is moxibustion, that is, the burning of moxa. Schnorrenberger argues that the traditional Chinese name of acupuncture is *Chen-Chiu* ("penetration of the skin with needles and use of moxibustion"), which underlines the importance of this practice.[24] Moxa is a little heap of dried and crushed leaves of mugwort (*Artemisia vulgaris*), which is placed on a certain point of acupuncture. It can be placed directly on the skin, on a slice of ginger, on the end of a special needle, in a burning container, or it can be compressed into a stick, which is set alight and held just above the acupuncture point. Another, more recent, practice, is electro-acupuncture, in which a low-intensity current is applied to the needles in order to stimulate the meridians even more.

Treatment consists of stimulation, or increase of *Chi* energy, if its level is too low in a meridian, or of dispersion of the excess *Chi* energy if its level is too high. The acupuncturist knows that there is a precise timetable for the flow of energy through the meridians, and that in each of the twelve meridians the *Chi* energy attains a maximum for two hours per day. During these two hours the acupuncturist can intervene with highest efficiency for dispersing energy in that meridian if it is in excess, and the next two hours are ideal for stimulating that meridian if *Chi* energy is deficient.

Excess of energy or its insufficiency in the principal meridians also affects one's mental states and even one's dreams. For example, excess energy in the liver meridian produces anger, while its insufficiency causes fear; excess in the kidneys produces dreams in which one finds it difficult to unfasten his belt, while insufficiency in the kidney meridian produces indecision, confused speech, and "dreams of inundated trees." Excess in the gallbladder causes excessive sleeping, while insufficiency produces insomnia; excess of energy in the urinary bladder produces "painful head when defecating," while insufficiency causes the thriving of intestinal worms.[25] If one dreams about wading "through a large body of water with fear and anxiety" or about "bamboo submerged in water," it means energy shortage in the kidneys; dreams of "mountains that burn, fire, smoke" speak of emptiness of the heart; dreams of "uncultivated fields and countryside" speak of insufficient energy in the large intestine, while dreams in which

---

24. Schnorrenberger, *Chen-Chiu*, 22.
25. Morant, *Chinese Acupuncture*, 98–99.

appear "marvelous objects of gold or iron" indicate insufficient energy in the lung.[26] All these clues are gathered in an interview in order to reach a precise diagnosis of one's real health condition.

As we can see, there is no relationship between the principles of reaching a diagnosis in Western medicine and those of acupuncture. While the brain is missing from the list of the principal organs of the body, the gallbladder and the spleen are among them, although they can be removed in extreme situations without endangering the patient's life. According to Chinese medicine, the consequences of cholecystectomy (the surgical removal of the gallbladder) or splenectomy (removal of the spleen) should be catastrophic on the patient's health. Morant states:

> The gallbladder has an important psychological action, unnoticed in Europe. Courage, audacity, intrepitude, timorousness and combativeness are proportional to its activity and fullness. Consequently, in Chinese, the most intrepid and combative soldiers are called the "grand gallbladders" (*da dan*). It is the organ of courage and combativeness (as the kidney is the organ of character and shrewdness, and the spleen-pancreas of intellectuality).[27]

Modern acupuncturists argue that in the case of a surgical removal of gallbladder or spleen we do not see the psychological impact we should expect, because although the physical organ is removed, its meridian remains. But if the energy channel and its well-being is all that matters, why do acupuncturists still need to formulate a close connection between energy flow in the meridians and physical organs, and why does not the entire healing technique of acupuncture become a philosophy completely detached from the physical body? In other words, if the link between the anatomy of acupuncture and that of Western medicine is weakened whenever acupuncture contradicts medical science, why should we not sever them completely from each other? Acupuncture and Western medicine work on fundamentally different premises, and Morant makes this point very clear:

> The pasteurian diagnosis, which defines an exterior entity, a microbe to fight, does not exist in energy. It is replaced by the measure of the intensity of the energy, either total, multiple, or local,

---

26. Morant, *Chinese Acupuncture*, 629–30.
27. Morant, *Chinese Acupuncture*, 134.; see also Mole, *Acupuncture*, 43.

by the radial pulses – the potential of the vitality of the subject. Where the energy is in balanced fullness, the microbe dies.[28]

6.5 HUMAN PHYSIOLOGY AND THE FIVE FUNDAMENTAL ELEMENTS

Since each meridian receives *Chi* energy from the one that precedes it, according to a precise timetable, the relationship between the correspondent organs is called "mother-son,"[29] which means that the "mother" meridian transmits *Chi* energy to the "son" meridian. According to this relationship, in the case of *yin* organs, the heart is the mother of the spleen, the spleen is the mother of the lung, the lung of the kidney, the kidney of the liver, and the liver is the mother of the heart. Therefore, when an organ has too little energy, the "mother" organ must be stimulated "to feed the son." If it has too much, the energy of the "son" organ must be dispersed, "to make the son 'hungry' and suck more energy from the mother."[30] As a concrete example, Morant affirms that "if the heart is weak, one must tonify its mother: the liver. If it is over-excited or painful, one must disperse its child: the spleen-pancreas (which in the daily flow of energy precedes the heart)."[31]

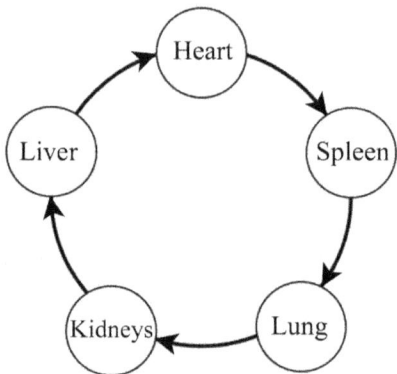

The mother-son relationship between the five *yin* organs

---

28. Morant, *Chinese Acupuncture*, 294. However, Pasteur's contribution to medicine is not ignored by modern acupuncturists, for they use disposable needles.
29. Morant, *Chinese Acupuncture*, 120.
30. Morant, *Chinese Acupuncture*, 120.
31. Morant, *Chinese Acupuncture*, 123.

Acupuncture and the Principles of Traditional Chinese Medicine

A second kind of relationship that exists between the organs is called of domination, or "the husband-wife rule," and is depicted in the next diagram. Domination relationships between *yin* organs are formulated as follows: the heart dominates the lung, the lung dominates the liver, the liver dominates the spleen, the spleen dominates the kidneys, and the kidneys dominate the heart. For example, Morant affirms that, "if the liver is ill, it will give the illness to the spleen-pancreas. In this case, the sage who cures what is not yet ill gives fullness of energy to the spleen-pancreas so that it does not receive the illness of the liver."[32]

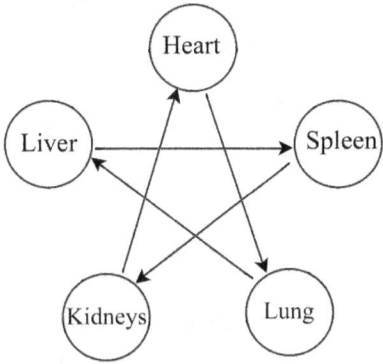

The husband-wife rule between the five *yin* organs

Since Chinese and modern medicine are so different, the question naturally arises: On what basis does Chinese medicine still work and yield results? What is the logic of its vision of the interaction between organs, that is, of the mother-son relationship and of the husband-wife rule? The answer comes from Taoism, the Chinese religion that lies at the foundation of acupuncture as a medical practice. According to a Taoist worldview, the relationship between organs corresponds to the relationship which exists between the five fundamental elements of Chinese cosmology (fire, earth, metal, water, and wood). These interact according to the mother-son relationship and the husband-wife rule: Fire generates earth (as ashes), earth produces metal (from ore), metal creates water (because dew condenses on metallic surfaces), water creates wood (by feeding vegetation), and wood creates fire (by combustion). The husband-wife rule works between the fundamental elements following the arrows in the next diagram: fire controls

32. Morant, *Chinese Acupuncture*, 122.

metal (by melting it), metal controls wood (an iron saw cuts wood), wood controls earth (the plant rises out of the ground and cracks it), earth controls water (sets the boundaries of the rivers and seas, absorbs water after it rains), and water controls fire (by extinguishing it). This is the rationale that inspires the relationship between body organs in acupuncture.

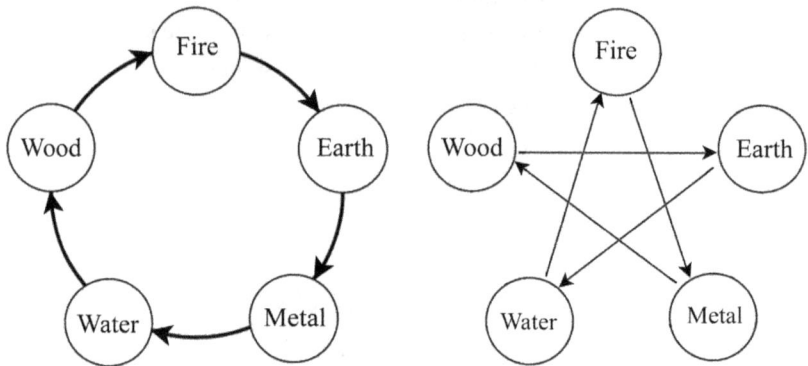

Mother-son and husband-wife relationships between elements

Only as a result of associating body organs with fundamental elements of Chinese cosmology can we understand the mother-son relationship between organs, that is, why the heart upholds the spleen, why the spleen feeds the lung, why the liver must be invigorated in order to strengthen the heart, and so on. The relationship between fundamental elements is the key for understanding the mother-son relationship and the husband-wife rule, and how illness is transmitted from one organ to the other. Since water extinguishes fire, the kidneys can transmit their illness to the heart, so the heart needs to be strengthened in the case of a kidney illness. Since metal cuts wood, the lungs can transmit their illness to the liver, so the liver must be fortified in case of a lung illness. Earth sets the borders of rivers and seas, therefore the spleen affects the kidneys, and because wood covers the earth, we can expect that the liver will transmit its disease to the spleen, and so on.

Taoists had no problem connecting the mother-son relationship and the husband-wife rule to their medical views. This is why acupuncture works best within a Taoist framework, and delivers the best results when one accepts the religious system as a whole. For this same reason, Western acupuncturists with no religious basis in Taoism have little results compared to Chinese practitioners who are accustomed to these beliefs and to the whole *Chi*-energy mechanisms that rule the world. A couple of French acupuncturists confirm this close relationship to Taoist beliefs, when they affirm that "all acupuncture and its associated therapies: moxibustion and Chinese massage, cannot be studied without knowing a particular conception of human physiology and its relationship with the organization of the universe."[33]

Chinese acupuncturists know how to take the pulses, interpret organ interactions according to the above mentioned rules, examine the patient's secretions, odors, tastes, and sounds. They do not simply use the diagnosis established by a medical practitioner, and then search for the acupuncture points in a manual.[34] Only the careful examination of pulses and all other clues discovered by following the ancient rules will reveal the correct diagnosis, as a local imbalance of energy. Since very long training is needed, Morant criticizes Western practitioners for their superficial approach:

> The pulses give a clear indication of the functioning, vitality, and energetic capacity of each internal organ; moreover, they inform us about the material form of the organ, be it large or small, hard or soft. The pathological state to be discerned necessitates such a delicacy of digital and cerebral perception that Europeans rarely succeed in perceiving it.[35]

6.6 ACUPUNCTURE AND CHRISTIANITY

Western practitioners often encourage the use of acupuncture without adopting its spiritual ground, suggesting that the wise men of ancient China discovered many secrets of the human body, but naturally formulated medical practice according to the religious views of their time. They assume that acupuncture has a scientific basis, but it has not yet been discovered. However, this "not yet" strategy is baseless. On the one hand, "modern" acupuncturists who reject its religious grounds have little success in medical practice.[36] Those who hold a certificate in acupuncture after

---

33. Guillaume et al., *L'acupuncture*, 21.

34. Morant argues: "The knowledge of pulses is absolutely indispensable for the practice of true acupuncture, which is based on treating the root condition. Using only memorized formulae and treating only visible problems does not constitute true acupuncture" (*Chinese Acupuncture*, 56).

35. Morant, *Chinese Acupuncture*, 56.

36. For an in-depth investigation of the success of acupuncture see Singh and Ernst, *Trick or Treatment?* In this book you can find a scientific study of the placebo effect (pp.

graduating a crash-course, but are unable to take the pulses, to interpret the smell of a patient's breath, sweat, urine, stools, and genital secretions, and are incapable of integrating all this "strange" information into a Taoist worldview, are not true acupuncturists, and their practice fails to produce notable results.

On the other hand, successful acupuncturists refuse to replace Taoist spiritual teachings with a scientific approach. They evaluate a patient as a little universe governed by laws other than those of science. Peter Mole, the Dean of the College of Integrated Chinese Medicine in Reading, UK, states that "any person who professes acupuncture without having studied Chinese medical theory and who maintains that it can be used as adjunct to Western medicine has failed to grasp its essence."[37] He rejects the "scientific" approach of finding acupuncture points with an instrument called a punctoscope, which measures the electrical conductivity of the skin, and of accepting diagnostics issued by Western medical doctors. This "scientific" approach does not bring the expected results.[38] Schnorrenberger holds that "its astonishing efficacy is only manifested when the practitioner adheres to the original teachings worked out thousands of years ago."[39] That is why "everywhere in the West where an attempt has been made to put *Chen-Chiu* on a "scientific" footing by subjecting it to the principles of Western natural science along the lines of the theoretical and methodical—to dissection and dismemberment—the result is always the opposite of that intended."[40]

Therefore there is no hope that sometime in the future the Taoist spiritual grounds of acupuncture will be replaced with new discoveries in modern medicine. Between the rationale of classical medicine and that of acupuncture there remains an insurmountable gap.

Hence we reach the unavoidable question: Can a Christian use acupuncture? As a practitioner, the rate of success depends on how much of its traditional religious views one absorbs. This is where problems start for a Christian, for the flow of *Chi* through our body is an automatism that needs to be understood and followed, an impersonal process that does not depend on a Creator God. The God of Christianity cannot be seen as two equal and opposite forces whose balance governs the world. God and

---

55–69) and an overall scientific assessment of acupuncture (pp. 69–88).

37. Mole, *Acupuncture*, 4.
38. Mole, *Acupuncture*, 13–14.
39. Schnorrenberger, *Chen-Chiu*, 81.
40. Schnorrenberger, *Chen-Chiu*, 85.

his angels, on the one side, and demons, on the other side, are indeed two opposite spiritual worlds, but they are not impersonal, nor equal, nor is the "negative force" everlasting. The fallen angels cannot be equated with a necessary *yin* force that balances the equilibrium in the spiritual world. Besides this important aspect, the world is not upheld by a kind of energy, such as *Chi*, but by God, a personal being, by his grace. As a result, we are not mere energy circuits that need to remain in harmony with the grand circuit of the entire universe, but persons meant for personal and everlasting communion with the Holy Trinity.

Therefore a "Christian" acupuncturist can either ignore the spiritual grounds of this art of healing, and then have no significant results in his or her practice, or be a successful healer, but ignore Christian teachings. As patients, Christians usually employ acupuncture either because they have little information about its spiritual ground, believing it is a kind of nerve stimulation that science has not yet been able to explain, or because, in search for healing at any price, they simply do not care about its mechanisms. As such, they may experience some improvement and become curious about what has actually healed them. Then they start to learn its underlying spirituality. If health is more important than their faith, they are slowly drawn towards beliefs that will weaken their faith, or even reach the point where it will crumble completely.

7

Reflexology

THE WORKING PRINCIPLES OF acupuncture can be found in other forms of alternative medicine as well. In pressopuncture (or acupressure) the healer restores the energy balance by pressing the acupuncture points with the fingers instead of using needles. Shiatsu (of Japanese origin) combines pressopuncture with massaging the meridians by using the palms, elbows, knees, or even soles. Another technique, which is halfway between acupuncture and reflexology, is auricular acupuncture (or ear acupuncture). It works on the assumption that all body organs are represented on the ears, following a chart which represents the whole body as a curled fetus (head down and oriented backwards). The needles are inserted into points of the ear corresponding to the internal organs, the effects being similar to those of classical acupuncture.

This way of representing the body organs in distant parts of the body is called zone theory. It defines reflex zones as precise locations on the body that correspond to internal organs, sense organs, or limbs, and whose stimulation triggers a response from the organs they represent. Barbara Kunz argues that zone theory is related to acupuncture, for "just as meridians link one part of the body with another, so a combination of zone charts and maps connects the hands and feet to the organs and structures of the body."[1] The best known form of alternative medicine based on zone theory is reflexology. In Louise Keet's definition,

> The theory underlying reflexology is that the organs, nerves, glands, and other parts of the body are connected to reflex areas

---

1. Kunz, *Complete Reflexology*, 22.

or reflex points on the feet and hands. These areas are found on the soles of the feet and palms of the hands, as well as on the top and sides of the feet and hands. By stimulating these areas using a compression technique and a form of massage with your thumbs, fingers and hands, you can create a direct response in a related body area.[2]

Most reflex zones are represented on the sole, but some are on the upper side of the foot, on the sides, and above the ankle. The same reflex zones are represented on the hands, but their use is considered less effective. On the surface of the sole three areas are defined: the front third of the sole corresponds to the organs above the diaphragm (the head, neck, heart, and lungs), the middle third corresponds to organs situated above the waist (for example, the stomach, liver, and kidneys), and the back third (the heel) corresponds to organs below the waist line (for example, the feet and sexual organs).

There are two major theories that try to explain how reflexology works, as well as attempts to find a middle ground between them. The first avoids spiritual teachings inspired from Taoism or other religions, and tries to define reflexology within the limits of a biological, not yet discovered, mechanism, while the second is heavily indebted to the views of Eastern religions. In order to distinguish them I will call the first physical reflexology, and the second spiritual reflexology.

7.1 PHYSICAL REFLEXOLOGY

The first form, seemingly unrelated to Eastern thought, affirms that diseases can be diagnosed and treated by massaging reflex zones on the foot or hand, assuming that in those zones deposits of crystals have formed that obstruct the blood flow, and thus the organs represented in these zones are affected. As Keet explains:

> A reflexologist discovers congested areas by finding crystals in the feet. These crystals are made up of uric acid or calcium and build up in the nerve endings in the feet. (. . .) By applying pressure to these crystals, the reflexologist will break them up, so that they dissolve and are carried away in the blood. The more crystals you

---

2. Keet, *The Reflexology Bible*, 8–10.

find, the longer you should work on them, so that they can be broken down by reflexology.³

However, there is no scientific confirmation that such crystal deposits exist in the alleged reflex zones, for it is only the reflexologist who claims to sense them and to have them removed by massage. Another attempted explanation, which does not mention such deposits in the soles, assumes that reflexology is a way of stimulating nerves linked to the respective organs. If this were the case, however, we should observe grave effects on organs when their reflex zones are injured, for instance by accidentally stepping on a sharp nail.⁴ So the nerve correspondence claim lacks scientific confirmation.

Since there is no medical confirmation of how physical reflexology works, its practitioners are very careful when making claims of its success. Joan Cosway-Hayes affirms it has three simple principles of action: reducing body tension and congestion, improving blood and lymph circulation, as well as oxygen flow, and normalizing body functions.⁵ She clearly states that "the reflexologist is not allowed to make *any* claims for reflexology," that is, "to say that reflexology will improve any specific condition."⁶ In her view, the reflexologist must not substitute the medical doctor, does not issue a diagnosis based on what he or she senses on the soles, and does not prescribe treatments, for "diagnosing, prescribing and treating all come under the realm of the medical doctor."⁷ What a reflexologist *can* claim, is that this technique can release body tension, improve circulation, and help body processes to normalize.

Apart from the massage itself, most practitioners of physical reflexology associate it with phytotherapy⁸ and a diet based on fresh fruit, veg-

---

3. Keet, *The Reflexology Bible*, 50.

4. For example, why is there no effect on the heart when one accidentally steps on a sharp nail and it pierces right through the heart zone?

5. Cosway-Hayes, *Reflexology for Every Body*, 13.

6. Cosway-Hayes, *Reflexology for Every Body*, 13.

7. Cosway-Hayes, *Reflexology for Every Body*, 13.

8. Phytotherapy is the use of medication produced from raw plants, mostly as tea, cataplasms, or tinctures. Although it originates in folk tradition, phytotherapy is rather a form of evidence-based medicine than one of the forms of alternative medicine analyzed in this book. For instance, St. John's wort (*Hypericum perforatum*) tea is good for heartburn (and I use it as such), not because of "profound spiritual principles" involved, but simply because it neutralizes the excess of acid produced by the stomach.

etables, and honey. Therefore, when patients feel an improvement in their condition, what did really help? Massage for removing "crystals," stimulating blood circulation by massage, the diet associated with this practice, phytotherapy, or the psychotherapy session that the healer offers during massage? Maybe all of them contribute, so there is no need for recourse to explanations involving *Chi* energy balancing. Massage itself has an obvious refreshing effect, which I personally experienced during a reflexology session, without having suffered any particular illness.

7.2 A LARGE VARIETY OF REFLEXOLOGY FORMS

As we have seen so far, classic reflexology affirms the representation of the body organs in the soles and palms, while auricular reflexology focuses on the ears. There are several other forms of reflexology, which define different reflex zones. In craniosacral reflexology the reflex zones on the feet are said to act upon the cranial nerves and the cerebro-spinal fluid. Spinal column reflexology (not to be mistaken for osteopathy or chiropractic) defines reflex zones at the tips of the vertebrae. Each vertebra corresponds to a certain organ or part of the body, so treatment consists of gentle tapping on the vertebral apophysis with the fingers or by exerting pressure on it.

In addition, there are at least two forms of reflexology of Eastern origin: Vietnamese facial reflexology (*Dien Chan*) and the Korean fingers and toes reflexology (*Su Jok*). The former was brought to the West by the Vietnamese master Bui Quôc Châu, who found his inspiration in sources such as Zen Buddhism, Taoism, Confucianism, I Ching, and Vietnamese folk tradition. Vietnamese facial reflexology works on the assumption that the reflex zones are located on the face,[9] but unlike other variants of reflexology, it considers that "the projections and points on the face are not a direct link to the physical body but to the brain," and thus the skin is "seen as a relay to the brain activating the process of self healing."[10]

---

9. *Dien* means "face," while *Chan* means "treatment and diagnostic."

10. Hilarius-Ford, *Origins and development of Facial Reflexology*, online. This form includes the belief that *Chi* energy flow is associated with healing, claiming that "the stimulation of the zones or points activates the process of self-regulation in the corresponding organ in the brain that guides our vital energy Qi to the corresponding affected zone" (same source).

Korean reflexology *Su Jok*[11] uses two different correspondence systems. Both consider the fingers and toes to be the location of reflex zones. According to one system, called the *Main correspondence system*, "the thumb corresponds to the neck and head, the forefinger and the little finger – to the upper limbs, the middle and the fourth fingers – to the lower limbs and the palm (foot) – to the torso."[12] According to the other correspondence system, called the *Insect correspondence system*, any of the fingers can represent the entire body. For example, massaging the back of any finger will act on the spine. One can use a ring that is pressed and rotated up or down a finger to stimulate in turn all organs.

Given this large variety of reflexology forms, we might wonder how can all of them work, despite the differences in locating reflex zones. For example, what reflex zone should be used to alleviate back pain? The arch of the soles (according to classical reflexology), a different zone in the sole (according to craniosacral reflexology), the mid-ear cartilage (according to auricular reflexology), the apophysis of a vertebra (according to vertebral reflexology), a certain point on the face (according to *Dien Chan*), or a part of a finger (according to *Su Jok*)? Or all in turn? Can all these variants work, or is there the same placebo effect at work in all?

7.3 REFLEXOLOGY AS A WAY OF CHANNELING VITAL ENERGY

The second major form of reflexology works on the *Chi*-energy theory defined in traditional Chinese medicine, and follows principles of Taoism and other Eastern religions. Unlike in physical reflexology, the connections between organs and reflex zones are defined as vital energy channels, and health is a concept that includes the well-being of unseen spiritual bodies.

In this and the following two sections of this chapter I will analyze three such spiritual reflexology forms, each with its own spiritual assumptions. These examples should serve as a warning for Christians that reflexology can be "spiritualized" and, although it seems to be nothing but a harmless therapy, or a simple way of inducing relaxation, it can still lead one to embrace spiritual views antithetical to Christianity.

Madeleine Turgeon, a Canadian reflexologist, is the first example. She follows closely on Taoist beliefs, arguing that "without knowing the

---

11. In Korean, *Su* is *hand*, and *Jok* is *foot*.
12. Mediks Ltd, "How does SU JOK heal," online.

principles of universal order, it is impossible to reach a good state of health, peace, justice, and happiness."[13] She allegedly finds these principles "of universal order" in the very first chapter of Genesis. But contrary to traditional Christianity, she interprets the creation account as meaning that "the One infinite polarized into two complementary and antagonistic forces: one positive and one negative,"[14] which is a reference to the *yin-yang* polarities. Such Taoist beliefs define the essence of her practice, and make it a close equivalent of acupuncture. In her words, "these two techniques are intimately linked by their common goal: to restore the balance of vital energy in the body."[15]

Turgeon's view of human nature is that of an energy circuit that needs to be balanced by pressing the reflex zones: "By allowing you to press the reflex buttons on the feet, hands and face, reflexology facilitates the distribution of vital energy in all your glands, organs, and your nervous system."[16] In other words, we resemble a battery which is more or less depleted and needs to be recharged: "The body is a system that functions like a battery, by ionic transfer from the healthy part to the injured part, as if electrical power would go to help the troubled part."[17] Given this view of human nature, the aim of reflexology is to restore the optimal working condition of this "battery," by reestablishing "the balance of vital energy to all glands and organs of the body."[18] If the energy flow is not balanced, the physical body will develop an organic illness, according to a general principle that we have already met, which says that "health problems are first – and almost always – energy based and functional before they become organic."[19]

Diseases are thus produced by energy imbalances, not by crystal deposits in the soles, so reflexology is a technique of transmitting *Chi* energy from a donor to a receiver. The donor is the reflexologist, who must

---

13. Turgeon, *Energie et réflexologie* [*Energy and reflexology*], 19.

14. Turgeon, *Energie et réflexologie*, 20.

15. Turgeon, *Découvrons la réflexologie* [*Discovering Reflexology*], 26. In an attempt to validate scientifically the existence of meridians and massage points in both acupuncture and reflexology, Turgeon mentions the Kirlian effect which would prove "the Chinese concept of vital energy circulating through the body on well-defined channels called meridians" (Turgeon, *Découvrons la réflexologie*, 26.). But as we have already seen in the chapter on Reiki, the Kirlian effect does not confirm any of this.

16. Turgeon, *Découvrons la réflexologie*, 27.

17. Turgeon, *Découvrons la réflexologie*, 39.

18. Turgeon, *Energie et réflexologie*, 42.

19. Turgeon, *Energie et réflexologie*, 66.

"concentrate his or her energy in the *Hara*,"[20] while the receiver is the patient, who lacks this energy and the skills to use it. In a way that reminds us of the handling of energy in Reiki, Turgeon argues that the healer must acknowledge that he or she is a mere "instrument in the service of universal energy, not the source of the energy itself,"[21] and "must have confidence in the energy, which knows how to guide itself."[22]

Christians are reassured that this energy-based view of human nature is consistent with their faith, since God created us like this: "These magical buttons are waiting patiently to be pressed in order to give you abundant physical energy, radiant health, a body without pain, and long-lasting youth, as the Creator intended."[23] In Turgeon's view, Jesus himself was a healer who mastered the flow of energy. He was one "who came the closest to a perfect knowledge of the mechanisms of the universe," but he was not unique among healers, since "most of the healing techniques used by Jesus and his disciples were already used in the ancient Far East."[24]

The view that Jesus was a skilled master who knew how to direct the flow of healing energy to ill people is also expressed by Reiki healers. However, this view distorts both his identity as the Son of God incarnate and the meaning of his way of healing people. As mentioned in the chapter on Reiki, Jesus healed people by his words, as a result of being the very Word of God, not by mastering *Chi* energy. Turgeon's view of Jesus and healing is significantly different from Christian teaching, for her sources of inspiration, as she confesses, were Taoism, tarot cards readings, and other divination methods such as I Ching and numerology.[25] However, as we have seen so far, from such sources cannot flow views on spirituality and healing consistent with Christianity.

---

20. Turgeon, *Energie et réflexologie*, 44. *Hara* is the Japanese name for the *dantien* of traditional Chinese medicine.

21. Turgeon, *Energie et réflexologie*, 52.

22. Turgeon, *Energie et réflexologie*, 53.

23. Turgeon, *Découvrons la réflexologie*, 27.

24. Turgeon, *Energie et réflexologie*, 25.

25. Turgeon, *Energie et réflexologie*, 19–26.

7.4 FROM REFLEXOLOGY TO A HINDU VIEW OF HUMAN NATURE

The next example of spiritual reflexology, in which we find a direct bridge from reflexology to Hindu spirituality, is that of the English reflexologist Pauline Wills. In her view,

> Disease starts in the aura, caused by blockages in this energy flow. If these diseases are not cleared, then the disease manifests in the physical body.[26]

The aura is the unseen part of our nature, which is composed of six "auric" bodies: the spiritual, causal, higher mental, mental, astral, and etheric. They can be imagined as concentric layers, from the outer physical and visible one, to the most important, which is the "essence of our being," that is, the spiritual body, called "the divine spark which is part of that ultimate reality or universal consciousness."[27] We can easily recognize here the self (*atman*) of Hinduism, the so-called divine core of our being. The causal body has the same role as in Hinduism, of a deposit that stores karma and lets it manifest in further lives. The higher mental body is "where inspirations and knowledge from the higher self manifest,"[28] the lower mental body is the seat of thoughts, while the astral body is that of emotions. The etheric body is composed of the seven *chakras* and the *nadis*, the channels through which *prana* flows.

According to Wills, reflexology "teaches that a vital energy called life force or prana circulates in a balanced rhythmic way between all the organs of the body. (. . .) If this energy becomes blocked, the organ relating to the blockage becomes dis-eased."[29] The role of the reflexologist, in her view, is to channel vital energy to the patient, in a way that reminds us of Reiki:

> When working on the feet of a patient, we should allow healing energy to flow through us, into our hands and into the patient. The energy of the earth comes through our feet. The energy of the universe flows through our crown chakra and both of these energies meet in the heart centre where they are united in love.

---

26. Wills, *Reflexology*, 8.
27. Wills, *Reflexology*, 9.
28. Wills, *Reflexology*, 9.
29. Wills, *Reflexology*, 35.

From the heart this energy flows through our arms and into our hands and fingers.[30]

The soles have reflex zones not only for physical organs, but also for the *chakras*, so they can be directly stimulated through massage. Another novelty of her healing technique is associating reflexology with color therapy, on the assumption that to each *chakra* corresponds a certain color, and by using light of that color one can improve the energy balance of that *chakra*. She presents two ways of using colors in therapy. One is mental, by visualizing a color and channeling it to the patient's *chakra*, and the other is physical, by using a special torch that projects a certain color on the reflex zone of the corresponding *chakra*.[31] For example, blue is the right color to deal with high blood pressure, so she would project blue light over the reflex zone of the heart *chakra*.[32]

In a similar way to Chopra, Wills upholds a close relationship between physical health, provided by the right functioning of the *chakras*, and religious liberation, achieved through the rise of *kundalini* through the very same *chakras*. She argues that the right functioning of the *chakras* is essential for two reasons. On the one hand, each *chakra* feeds energy to a group of organs and mental functions. On the other hand, the *chakras* are located along the *sushumna* channel and must stay open to allow *kundalini* to pass on its way to liberation. In order to achieve liberation, which should be one's ultimate goal, Wills faithfully follows Hindu teachings, indicating the mantras necessary for the opening of each *chakra* and the governing Hindu deities that need to be invoked.[33] On the importance of the last *chakra* she says: "This chakra leads us into the eternal, infinite, supreme existence. It is the centre of pure consciousness and the abode of Shiva. When the kundalini rises, Shiva and Shakti are united, bringing about a transformation in human consciousness," and one no longer needs "to reincarnate into a physical body."[34]

Such views could be part of a Hatha Yoga manual rather than of a book on reflexology. The reason for such a close symbiosis between spiritual liberation and health is that one must seek a much deeper sense of healing than just the physical.

30. Wills, *Reflexology*, 44.
31. Wills, *Reflexology*, 57.
32. Wills, *Reflexology*, 57.
33. Wills, *Reflexology*, 13–27.
34. Wills, *Reflexology*, 26–27.

Reflexology

The role of the healer is to be an instrument through which energy flows to the patient. In order to better fulfill this role, she prays for help to spiritual beings:

> Before the first patient of the day arrives, I always light a candle asking that I may be a channel through which the healing power of the universe flows. This candle can represent the Christ light, the Buddha light or the pure universal light.[35]

Unlike in other forms of reflexology, it is not enough to know how *Chi* works, or to find the proper balance of energy in oneself. Wills invites us to take a step further, to contact the spiritual beings who direct this energy, that is, to "acknowledge and work with the elementals who are responsible for the elements of earth, water, fire and air," and to "thank them for the tasks they are accomplishing."[36] As if reflexology becomes a kind of magic, these elementals must be treated with respect and fear. Wills affirms: "If we ask their help and thank them for helping us, they will become our friends and servants. If we misuse them, they can create havoc."[37]

Pauline Wills is a second example which shows how an apparently harmless form of alternative medicine can take one into spiritual realms alien to Christianity. Her spiritual views make it impossible for her to be, as she claims, an instrument of the "Christ light."[38] Using the name of Christ for promoting views opposed to Christian teachings can by no means make her use of reflexology acceptable for Christians.

7.5 FROM REFLEXOLOGY TO TIBETAN BUDDHISM

Another English reflexologist who has created a bridge from a simple sole massage technique to an Eastern religion, this time Tibetan Buddhism, is David Vennells. Having been healed of chronic fatigue syndrome by reflexology, Vennells decided to start practicing it himself.[39] He explains reflexology by combining the belief that there are nerve connections between reflex zones in the soles and body organs with traditional Chinese

---

35. Wills, *Reflexology*, 39.
36. Wills, *Reflexology*, 80.
37. Wills, *Reflexology*, 80.
38. Wills, *Reflexology*, 39, 93.
39. Reiki and Bach floral remedies also contributed to his healing (Vennells, *Reflexology*, xvii–xviii).

medicine and its way of explaining illness as the result of *Chi* energy blockages.[40] Shortly after starting his reflexology practice he discovered Tibetan Buddhism and understood that his patients needed a deeper healing than physical. His religious conversion gave him a new understanding of how the human mind works and allegedly led to better results in the practice of reflexology.[41] This new understanding, however, was not a new knowledge of brain physiology or psychology, but the result of following the spiritual practice of Tibetan Buddhism. Thus understanding Vennells's approach to reflexology will require a brief introduction to the Buddhist view on human nature.

Buddhism is based on three fundamental doctrines: impermanence, denial of a self, and suffering. The doctrine of impermanence (*anitya*) states that everything is permanently subjected to change, that nothing escapes the cycle of perpetual transformation, not even what religions call their ultimate reality. The consequence is that Buddhism categorically rejects the affirmation of any kind of ultimate reality, including the Christian view of God. The only "permanent" *something* is not a substance or a Person, but a truth, that of impermanence. The second doctrine, which follows logically from the first, is the denial of a self as stated in Hinduism. Therefore there is no "divine spark" or unchangeable substance in human nature that is reincarnated. What is reborn in Buddhism is not a "self," but only karma, which travels from one lifetime to the next as the flow of mental imprints, without the need of a substantial support. The third doctrine is that of suffering (*dukkha*), which is the result of the first two, affirming that human existence is wholly marked by suffering. Personal existence itself means suffering because we crave for stability, for an everlasting soul, and for stable relationships with God and our neighbors, which are all illusions.

According to Buddhist teaching, the "soul" is an illusion generated by five interlinked factors called aggregates (*skandha*): form (*rupa*), sensation (*vedana*), perception (*samjna*), volition (*samskarah*), and consciousness (*vijnana*). *Form* is the body with its six sense organs.[42] The senses generate *sensations* of pleasure, aversion or indifference. The process of organizing and labeling them into categories is called *perception*. As a result, *volitional*

40. Vennells, *Reflexology*, 6–7. However, he admits that "there is no definite evidence that makes it a conclusive, accurate, and definite theory" (Vennells, *Reflexology*, 7.).

41. Vennells, *Reflexology*, xx.

42. There are six senses because the mind is also called a sense organ. It senses the world of ideas and thoughts, just as the other five sense the five aspects of the material world.

acts are initiated in response to the objects of sensory experience, which bear consequences in this and further lives. Finally, *consciousness* means being aware of ourselves as subjects who witness a series of perceptions and thoughts. Consciousness creates the belief that one is a distinct agent of cognition, that there is a soul that observes and responds to the objects of perception, when in fact it is only the end result of a process dependent on sensory input. As a result, liberation means breaking free from this illusion, following the understanding of things as they really are. It is the extinction of craving for personal existence. One of the characteristic elements of Tibetan Buddhism, to be added here, is the importance of compassion for the one who manages to know how things really are. Compassion (*karuna*) is defined as a commitment to help all beings trapped in ignorance to free themselves from it and reach liberation.

According to Vennells, Buddhism should be set as the spiritual foundation for anyone who wants to understand human nature and the meaning of life:

> If you ever wanted to know who you are, why you're here, and where you're going, simply pick up a good book on Buddhism. It will be a map of reality.[43]

From a Buddhist perspective, health must be considered from a much wider and deeper perspective than the well-being of the body. In Vennells's words, "we need to look deeper within the nature of the mind to discover the actual cause of illness."[44] As we might expect, the "deeper" cause of illness is karma. Therefore suffering must be viewed from a perspective that goes beyond the insignificant particularities of the present life:

> From Buddhism we know that the root causes of all our major and minor problems are our own previous negative actions of body, speech, and mind returning to us as illness, poverty, ignorance, or any other type of unpleasant experience. (. . .) We all have an infinite amount of accumulated karma, because we have had countless previous lives.[45]

---

43. Vennells, *Reflexology*, 185. Instead of acknowledging that Buddhism is a way of extinguishing personal existence, Vennells presents it as the fulfillment of our highest hopes for happiness: "In fact, all we really need is a happy mind. Understanding the true causes of happiness and suffering is right at the heart of Buddhist philosophy" (Vennells, *Reflexology*, 172.).

44. Vennells, *Reflexology*, 166.

45. Vennells, *Reflexology*, 177–79.

In a way similar to what we have seen in Reiki and in other forms of alternative medicine which speak of reincarnation, karma explains why some illnesses cannot be cured through reflexology, so we must accept failures "with a peaceful and patient mind."[46] One who is not healed needs to investigate the deeper cause of illness, which is the karma of past lives. By accepting the Buddhist way of seeing things, we reach a deeper happiness, that of nirvana. So we are in a win-win situation. Either are we healed of a particular illness by Vennells's form of reflexology, or, if not, we follow Buddhism and become wiser. True healing is to reach enlightenment, and the first step towards it is to give up clinging to personal existence:

> We have a strong sense of self, a strong sense that we truly exist, and that this self is the most important thing in the universe. The fact that we grasp at this sense of self, ego, or I, and believe it to truly exist, is the source of all our present and future problems.[47]

Patients who do not change their way of understanding life will further fuel karma, and just prolong physical and spiritual illness.[48]

As we can see, Vennells invites his patients to a much more profound journey than just finding physical healing. Starting with reflexology he reached a whole new way of understanding the meaning of life through the teachings of Tibetan Buddhism. This, however, cannot be a desirable goal, for Christianity does not teach us to be "healed" of personal existence itself, but calls us to the exact opposite. The "deepest" possible healing is the healing from sin, and it is attained in a personal relationship with God, the true and permanent ultimate reality.

Let us remember that Vennells started his spiritual journey by seeking healing for his chronic fatigue syndrome. This condition could have led him to find Christianity, but a friend led him on the Buddhist way. Instead of finding Jesus and eternal life in him, Vennells found the way to nirvana, to extinguishing the illusion that a personal destiny would make any sense. His case shows the importance of Christian testimony, of being ready to help those who suffer by being the instruments of God's grace in their lives.

---

46. Vennells, *Reflexology*, 180. He affirms: "Ultimately, we can only remove the true causes of illness by knowing, experiencing, and purifying our very subtle mind of all the potential seeds of illness planted or created by our own past negative actions in previous lives" (Vennells, *Reflexology*, 180).

47. Vennells, *Reflexology*, 184.

48. Vennells, *Reflexology*, 187.

It also speaks of the need to find a deeper healing than the physical, one that would heal the soul as well.

7.6 ADDENDUM. IRIDOLOGY

Iridology is a form of alternative medicine which claims that body organs are represented on the iris of the eye. To each segment of the iris a certain organ is assigned, and the particular shapes that are seen in that segment tell of the health of its corresponding organ. Iridology can be used only as a diagnostic tool, while the actual treatment is done by other forms of alternative medicine, such as homeopathy and phytotherapy.

The idea that the iris can signal the manifestation of illnesses is contradicted by science. After the age of ten months the iris image remains constant for the rest of our life. This fact is the basis of the most accurate method of identifying people, more accurate than fingerprinting, called Iris Recognition.[49] If a disease and its healing could be traced on the iris as a modification of its image, Iris Recognition would be worthless. Consequently, the scientific investigation of iridology as a diagnosis method has led to very discouraging results.[50]

Since iridology cannot identify diseases that appear for a time and then disappear, modern iridologists try to present their method as a way of diagnosing general dispositions or weaknesses of the body that remain constant throughout one's life. Bernard Jensen (1908–2001), one of the most respected figures in iridology, investigated over 300,000 patients in his 62 years of practice, and his iris-maps are still used today. He affirms that iridologists must refrain from naming specific illnesses, and instead limit themselves to observing general predispositions to diseases.[51] Following such a general assessment of one's predispositions, he proposes a diet that would strengthen the body against the manifestation of those potential illnesses.

A completely different view of iridology, which goes deep into Eastern spirituality and astrology, is the one advocated by the Italian Osvaldo

---

49. It affirms that the possibility of two people having an identical iris is $1:10^{78}$ (1 followed by 78 zeroes) and therefore is considered the safest biometric identification method. For more information see irisid.com.

50. Knipschild P., "Looking for gall bladder disease in the patient's iris," 1578–81. See also Münstedt et al., "Can iridology detect susceptibility to cancer?, 515–19.

51. Jensen and Bodeen, *Visions of Health*, 16.

Sponzili. His study of astrology led him to the belief that the moment of one's birth determines one's entire life, including the illnesses he or she will develop. In Sponzili's words, on the iris is "printed at birth the entire life of a person, as an astral map."[52] On this map we can read "periods of crisis one has been through or will endure, organs that are genetically weakened, and the age when these weaknesses can become risky."[53] His understanding of Hinduism led him to formulate a view on human nature resembling that of the Upanishads, expressed in "modern" terms:

> Human beings have a body of light that comes from the field of Pure Potentiality, from the Self. Before being born, human beings were part of the All, the non-polarized Universal Energy. One's entry into the polarized world takes place at birth when he or she breathes for the first time and connects to the cosmic rhythms and becomes an essential and determining element of the macro-microcosmic system.[54]

This is a way of expressing the identity of the self (*atman* in Hinduism, here the "body of light") with the ultimate reality (Brahman in Hinduism, here "Pure Potentiality"), and the need to return to oneness, a process that requires many lives. Reincarnation is an indisputable fact of spiritual evolution, in which the causal body imprints the past in a visible way, on the iris. In Sponzili's words, "the miasmatic energy that comes from previous reincarnations will remain printed from birth in the structure of the iris with its gaps and colors."[55]

The "astral map" of the iris speaks not only of one's diseases, but also of one's karma. In a similar way to Chopra's approach to Ayurveda, for Sponzili an illness is not only a problem of the physical body, but also a call towards liberation. Although he affirms that "disease becomes an unmatched opportunity that God has given us on the path of knowledge and research of our origins," [56] he means by it the rediscovery of our "body of light," our spiritual self. Obviously, this is a very awkward form of iridology, but one that can serve as a warning on how a form of alternative medicine can appropriate deep esoteric beliefs.

---

52. Sponzili, *Iniziazione all'Iridologia* [*Initiation in Iridology*], 7.
53. Sponzili, *Iniziazione all'Iridologia*, 7
54. Sponzili, *Iniziazione all'Iridologia*, 101.
55. Sponzili, *Iniziazione all'Iridologia*, 103.
56. Sponzili, *Iniziazione all'Iridologia*, 102.

8

Homeopathy

THIS IS PROBABLY THE most controversial of all forms of alternative medicine, partly because its esoteric aspect is hard to discern, and partly because it is very popular among Christians. Homeopaths present it as a science, similar to evidence-based medicine, whose success does not depend on the spiritual beliefs of those who use it. Its critics call it quackery, fake science, the reminiscence of pre-scientific vitalistic theories, and thus a waste of time and money. For homeopathy fans all that matters is that it heals; for its critics it can work only as a placebo effect. The controversy exists also among Christians, for many consider it a form of medicine that avoids antibiotics and other drugs, and cannot see in it anything that would compromise one's faith.

The one thing that is generally acknowledged about homeopathy is that it cannot be explained scientifically. But this argument by itself is not sufficient for Christians to reject homeopathy. Neither can faith be explained scientifically. A certain medical or pseudo-medical practice cannot be regarded as intrinsically evil just because we cannot understand its mechanisms on a scientific basis. The father of medicine, Hippocrates (c. 460 – c. 370 BC), was not a Christian, but a follower of the cult of Asclepius, the Greek god of medicine and healing. But that did not prevent him from establishing evidence-based medicine, that is, a careful observation of the symptoms and the effects of ancient treatments. Modern medicine does not work on the *religious* beliefs of Hippocrates, Pasteur or Fleming, but on the basis of scientific principles that operate regardless of the religious convictions of its founders. And between science and Christian faith there cannot be a genuine contradiction, since both have their source in God. As we have seen so far in this book, it is not the non-scientific content of a form of alternative medicine that makes it undesirable for Christians, but the fact that it involves spiritual concepts that distort or run counter to the content of our faith. This is what we need to discern in homeopathy.

8.1 SAMUEL HAHNEMANN

The founder of homeopathy is the German doctor Samuel Hahnemann (1755–1843). He was horrified by the medical practices of his time, such as "bloodletting in torrents," "starvation diet," leech therapy, enemas, and the use of drugs made of mercury, lead, arsenic, and poisonous plants, for they were doing more harm to patients than good.[1] He called this destructive medicine "the old school," and thought that "it was high time that the wise and benevolent Creator and Sustainer of humanity put a stop to these atrocities, bid these tortures cease, and brought a medical art to the light of day which is the opposite of all."[2] Modern doctors would probably agree with him given the horrors endured by the patients of his time. As such, the emergence of homeopathy was medical progress, even if based entirely on the placebo effect. Patients of those days would probably have done better if they received no treatment at all from the "old school" of medicine. But that does not mean that we should manifest the same horror for today's medicine.

Hahnemann studied medicine in Leipzig for two years, moved to Vienna for one year, worked as a librarian for the Count von Brukenthal for a year and a half (1777–79) in Hermannstadt (today's Sibiu, in Romania), and in 1779 returned to Germany and completed his medical studies at the University of Erlangen. During his stay in Hermannstadt he was initiated in Freemasonry, which raises many questions about his religious beliefs.[3]

---

1. *Organon*, 74. The principles of homeopathy are formulated by Hahnemann in the text-book of this practice, *Organon of the Medical Art*, which reached the fifth edition during his lifetime (1833). Quotes in this chapter belong to the final edition, the sixth, which was published posthumously. When quoting from the *Organon*, I will indicate only the number of the paragraphs (also called aphorisms).

2. *Organon*, "Introduction."

3. He was admitted to the first degree of the Masonic Lodge on October 16, 1777 (Haehl, *Samuel Hahnemann*, 10). In a letter he wrote at the age of 66, he reaffirmed his belonging to Freemasonry and his willingness to meet "true Masons" (Haehl, *Samuel Hahnemann*, 125).

Homeopathy

Since there is much speculation on this topic, I will confine myself to presenting objective data from his biography and letters. From the testimony of Ernst von Brunnow, one of his disciples, we find out that,

> With regard to religion, Hahnemann, who belonged to the Lutheran confession, held aloof from all dogmatic creeds. He was a pure Deist, but he was this with full conviction.[4]

Deism affirms the creation of the world by a divine being, to which we owe the order and logic of the world, but does not accept particular revelations, ascribing to reason the role of formulating the correct understanding of the world. This is the context in which we need to interpret some of Hahnemann's statements that seem to be consistent with Christianity, such as: "I cannot cease to praise and thank God when I contemplate his works."[5] He was grateful to this god of deism for the discovery of homeopathy, when he said it was "revealed to me by God, and I can acknowledge it with emotion and thankfulness."[6]

The discovery that made him famous came in 1790, as he translated a medical paper that discussed the newly discovered properties of quinine in treating malaria. He decided to try the effect of quinine on himself, although he was not suffering from malaria and, surprisingly, began to manifest the same symptoms that quinine can cure, that is, fever and chills. This led him to formulate the first principle of homeopathy, the Law of Similars—*similia similibus curentur*—that is, "let similar be cured by similar."[7] It means that a homeopathic remedy heals an illness whose symptoms are induced by that remedy in a healthy person. For example, as quinine induces the symptoms of malaria in a healthy person, it can cure the same symptoms, and the illness associated with them, in the case of an ill person. This first principle is the origin of its name, for in Greek, *homoios* means *the same*, and *pathos* means *suffering*. The "old school" of medicine was called *allopathy*, for it used medicines with effects *opposite* of the disease's symptoms.

In the years that followed, Hahnemann tested numerous remedies on himself, his family members, and students, carefully writing down all the

---

4. Bradford, *The Life and Letters*, 112.
5. Bradford, *The Life and Letters*, 112.
6. Bradford, *The Life and Letters*, 182.
7. This formula contains an imperative: "Let similar be cured by similars!" Therefore the often used formula, even by homeopaths—*similia similibus curantur* ("like is cured by like")—is not accurate.

symptoms they produced, of both a physical and a mental nature.[8] This collection of symptoms, continued by his followers, is the content of the treatise called *Homeopathic Materia Medica* ("the collected body of knowledge"). Another important tool he produced is the homeopathic repertory, a kind of index in which symptoms are associated with the right remedy for every illness. Remedies were prepared from plants, animals, or even minerals, synthetic chemicals, and products taken from diseased persons, such as urine, blood, or tissue.[9] The process of testing and noting the effects of each remedy is called "proving," and the subjects involved are "provers." For the most objective identification of the symptoms produced by his remedies Hahnemann used healthy people of different ages and of both sexes.

8.2 THE PREPARATION OF HOMEOPATHIC REMEDIES

Since many of the remedies are poisonous in raw form, Hahnemann had the intuition that they must be diluted as much as possible to achieve the best effect. This is the foundation of the second principle of homeopathy, that of the minimum dose, which requires the progressive dilution of homeopathic remedies. Paradoxically, instead of losing their healing power, as science would predict, dilution, as prescribed by Hahnemann, leads to a growth of their effectiveness.

The raw substances used for preparing remedies are in most cases plant tinctures, that is, alcohol extracts, in which a certain part of a plant (like its flowers) has been kept for several days. From such a tincture, one takes one part, adds 99 parts of the proper solvent,[10] the mixture is shaken vigorously and thus is obtained the first centesimal dilution (1:100), called C1. The shaking (called succussion) is not done randomly, but according to Hahnemann's instructions: "Give the tightly corked vial 100 strong succussions with the hand against a hard but elastic body."[11] Succussion, as-

---

8. For example, important clues can be found from the patient's behavior during sleep: "How does the patient gesticulate and express himself in his sleep? Does he whimper, groan, talk or cry out in his sleep? Does he get frightened during sleep? Does he snore on breathing in or breathing out?" (*Organon*, 89, footnote).

9. Such products are called *nosodes*. One contemporary extreme example of *nosodes* are bodily fluids from AIDS and Ebola victims, which obviously involves a dangerous procedure for obtaining remedies.

10. The solvent can be water, if the raw substance is soluble in water, or alcohol (45–65 percent).

11. *Organon*, 270.

Homeopathy

sociated with the progressive dilutions, is said to potentize (or dynamize) the healing powers of the initial substance, an aspect to which I will return.

Next, one takes one part of the C1 dilution, mixes it with another 99 parts of solvent, shakes it again, which results in the C2 dilution (or potency), and so on until very high dilutions are obtained. Centesimal dilutions are the most common, while decimal dilutions—noted by X (diluted 1:10, instead of 1:100) are less frequent.[12] If we apply what we were taught in high school chemistry and calculate the concentration of the remaining active substance in the homeopathic remedy, we will see that once the C12 or 24X dilution is reached, there is not one molecule of the active substance left in that homeopathic remedy.[13] Therefore, the progressive dilution process not only eliminates the toxicity of the initial raw substance, but all of it, in potencies that exceed C12.

When preparing remedies out of insoluble substances, such as pure gold (to obtain *Aurum Metallicum*) or chalk (to obtain *Calcium Carbonicum*), these are subjected to a process called trituration. This means mixing them with lactose (milk sugar) powder in a 1:100 ratio in a mortar, grinding the mixture with a pestle, and thus obtaining the equivalent of the C1 "dilution." Then one part is mixed with another 99 parts of lactose powder, and one gets the C2 dilution, and so on. At one point the solid powder is mixed with water in a 1:100 ratio and the process continues as above. The final dilution is impregnated in small sugar globules or stored as a solution. These are the remedies we find in homeopathic pharmacies.

According to homeopathic theory, the process of potentization explains why some remedies have no effect in a raw (initial) state. For instance, *Natrium Muriaticum* (salt) does not produce significant symptoms in its natural state (we all use it in preparing meals), but once it is diluted according to homeopathic procedure it produces strong symptoms. According to William Boericke's *Materia Medica*, these include:

---

12. Decimal dilutions were introduced by Hering (1800–1880). In his later years in Paris Hahnemann experimented much greater dilutions, of 1:50.000, which are noted LM or Q.

13. If you cannot remember this from chemistry class, Avogadro's number means that one mole of a substance contains 6.022×10^{23} particles. For instance 58.5 grams of salt (Sodium chloride) contain 6.022×10^{23} pairs of sodium and chloride ions (Na^+ and Cl^-). Although this number is astronomical, once the initial salt solution that is used to prepare *Natrium Muriaticum* is diluted twelve times in a 1:100 ratio (leading to the C12 potency) there is not a single ion left from the initial salt solution. Still, in homeopathy enormously high dilutions are used, as high as C100,000.

- (mental:) "grief, fright, anger, etc. Depressed, particularly in chronic diseases."
- (head symptoms:) "Aches as if a thousand little hammers were knocking on the brain, in the morning on awakening, *after menstruation*, from *sunrise* to *sunset*."
- (on the eyes:) "Letters run together. Sees sparks. Fiery, zigzag appearance around all objects."
- (respiratory:) "Cough from a tickling in the pit of stomach, accompanied by stitches in liver and spurting of urine. Stitches all over chest. Cough, with bursting pain in head. Shortness of breath, especially on going upstairs."
- (on the heart:) "Tachycardia. Sensation of coldness of heart. Heart and chest feel constricted. Fluttering, palpitating; intermittent pulse. Heart's pulsations shake body."
- (on sleep:) "Sleepy in forenoon. Nervous jerking during sleep. Dreams of robbers. Sleepless from grief."[14]

8.3 THE PERSONALIZATION OF TREATMENT

The third principle of homeopathy is the personalization of treatment, based on the belief that it is not the illness that needs to be treated, but the individual patient, whose illness has individual causes. Therefore, in order to find the proper remedy, the patient is subjected to a long and detailed interview in which not only his or her pains are assessed, but also a sum of more complex factors, such as "discernible body constitution, mental and emotional character, occupations, lifestyle and habits, civic and domestic relationships, age, sexual function, etc."[15] Here are some questions asked by the world leading Greek homeopath George Vithoulkas:

> Do you have any fears (of dogs, of the dark, of death, of closed places, of heights)? Are you anxious, and if so, over what kind of things (your health, other people)? Are you usually neat or sloppy? How are you affected by music? Are your complaints mostly on

---

14. Boericke, *Materia Medica*, online. Boericke (1849–1929) was one of the leading figures of homeopathy in the U.S., co-founder of the Pacific Homoeopathic Medical College and Hahnemann Hospital in San Francisco (1881).

15. *Organon*, 5.

one side of your body – which side? Do you have any particularly strong cravings or aversions for specific foods? How do you sleep? What position do you sleep in? Do you stick your feet out from under the covers?[16]

Hahnemann prescribed a single remedy at a time to a patient, depending on his or her particular constitution and symptoms, after which he expected to see the results, and then continued the treatment with the same remedy, in another potency, or with another remedy. This is the method called the *unicist* approach. More recently a new method of homeopathic treatment has emerged that simultaneously administers three or more remedies at a time. This is done for practical reasons, with the hope that the right one would be among them. This is the *pluralist* approach, which Hahnemann would have opposed vehemently, for it violates the fundamental laws of homeopathy.[17]

Hahnemann's observation that some diseases do not respond properly to his remedies led him to the conclusion that there are two kinds of diseases: acute and chronic. Acute diseases are easy to treat, while chronic diseases have a deeper cause. This "deeper cause," called a miasm, is harmful content we have inherited from our parents and accumulated in life.[18] It is a kind of weakness that is permanently carried by the individual and transmitted to his or her descendants as a debilitating condition that weakens the body and makes it prone to diseases.

The miasm can be of three kinds: psora, sycosis, and syphilis.[19] Psora is the most common. In Hahnemann's words, "Psora is the true *fundamental cause* and engenderer of almost all the other remaining forms of disease which are numerous, indeed countless."[20] While in Western medicine psora is seen as a skin disease (scabies), in homeopathy it is something much deeper; a fundamental breakdown that the body cannot defeat without the help of a homeopathic remedy. Psora, like the other two miasms, is identified on the basis of a careful observation of all physical and psychological symptoms of the patient, not just the aspect of itching

---

16. Vithoulkas, *Homeopathy: Medicine for the New Millennium*, 56.

17. *Organon*, 273.

18. *Miasma* is a concept that has existed since Hippocrates, referring to "morbific agents in the atmosphere, 'exhalations' from the soil causing epidemics" (Koehler, *The Handbook of Homeopathy*, 178).

19. *Organon*, 79.

20. *Organon*, 80.

skin. Itching is just one of the signs that indicate the presence of psora. In Hahnemann's view, psora produces a multitude of diseases, including mental disorders. In his list of diseases produced by psora we find "nervous debility, hysteria, hypochondria, mania, melancholia, imbecility, frenzy, epilepsy and convulsions of all kinds, bone-softening (rachitis), scrofula, scoliosis and kyphosis, bone caries, cancer, fungus hematodes, neoplasms, gout, hemorrhoids."[21]

James Tyler Kent (1849–1916), the second most important figure after Hahnemann and the father of modern homeopathy, continued this assessment of psora, affirming that "all the diseases of man are built upon psora."[22] Challenging what is today common knowledge in modern medicine, he states that "the five forms of Bright's disease are not diseases, but the result of psora operating upon the economy and attacking the kidney. The common chronic diseases of the liver are not diseases, but the localization of psora in the liver; the lung diseases and heart diseases and brain diseases are not diseases, because they have one single origin (which is psora)."[23]

Since a miasm is the deep cause of all illnesses, true healing means first of all overcoming the miasm and not just its manifestations, such as those of the skin. Otherwise a phenomenon called suppression will occur, that is, annihilating the symptoms, while the illness will only get worse over time. This is how the "old school" of medicine treats its patients; it only treats the symptoms, only the skin in the case of scabies, but leaves the fundamental problem unsolved.

The theory of miasms, however, raises a serious problem for the rationale of "proving," that is, the process of recording the symptoms caused by a remedy to a healthy person. The contradiction we are facing is raised by the fact that, in the words of Kent, "everyone is psoric."[24] Since *all* people have psora as a chronic disease, and all known diseases are just different

---

21. *Organon*, 80.
22. Kent, *Lectures*, 146.
23. Kent, *Lectures*, 153. Kent is the author of the *Repertory of the Homeopathic Materia Medica* (1897), which is used by homeopaths to this day. He died of Bright's disease at the age of 67.
24. Kent, *Lectures*, 156. Ann Jerome Croce confirms this belief among contemporary homeopaths: "Everyone has psora, but not everyone has the skin disease from which it originated; the same principle is true of the syphilitic miasm, which affects many people but very few of those affected have had the actual disease called syphilis" (online source: https://www.homeopathycenter.org/homeopathy-today/thought-behind-action-miasms-psora-syphilis-sycosis, retrieved December 13, 2019).

manifestations of it, *all* those who tested homeopathic remedies, including Hahnemann, have their nature affected by psora. As a result, they cannot be provers, that is, subjects that can provide objective symptoms of those remedies. If *all* people suffer from psora, Hahnemann's subjects were all ill and thus compromised the accuracy of the symptoms they described. The content of the *Materia Medica* is therefore rendered worthless. In other words, nobody is able to offer clear symptoms for a remedy, as prover, for all have psora, and as a result, there is no way of finding out what remedy should be given to an ill person.

8.4 HOMEOPATHY AND SCIENCE

Before assessing the spiritual side of homeopathy we need to understand that it has no scientific basis whatsoever.[25] At any rate no one so far has been able to formulate a convincing scientific explanation of how homeopathy works.[26] Here lies the paradox of this practice: It cannot be scientifically explained, but it nevertheless yields results. Otherwise it would have disappeared long ago.

Let us recall the facts that compromise any possible relationship between science and homeopathy. First of all, we need to know that although very low amounts (if anything) of a substance remain in a remedy, these remedies are not the equivalent of vaccines. In an attenuated vaccine a small amount of an attenuated virus exists, which causes the immune system to respond. In the case of homeopathy, most remedies no longer contain a single molecule of active substance, so they are not vaccines. For the same reason, homeopathy is not a form of phytotherapy. Phytotherapy uses plants in the form of teas, tinctures, cataplasms, baths, etc., in which the curative properties of plants are present as biochemical substances in a measurable quantity, whereas in homeopathy these substances have been lost completely, following dilution.

---

25. For a scientific investigation of homeopathy see Singh and Ernst, *Trick or Treatment?*, 36–62.

26. You will probably have heard of extravagant theories couched in scientific terms. For instance, Vithoulkas affirms that "We know from clinical results that the therapeutic energy still retains the 'vibrational frequency' of the initial substance," as if this would make any sense (Vithoulkas, *The Science of Homeopathy*, 104). However, two paragraphs later he leaves this complicated issue to future scientific investigation: "It will have to be left to physicists and chemists to discover precisely how energy is transferred to the solvent through this technique."

Second, I need to dispel the myth that homeopathic remedies function on the so-called water-memory effect. According to this theory, water molecules have the property of retaining the memory of substances they came in contact with, so during potentization a transfer of "information" takes place from the initial raw substance to the final remedy. This information is allegedly stored by the homeopathic remedy and used to induce healing. The hard part in this theory is to explain how the "information" held by the raw substance is kept by the water molecules. On the one hand, it is true that water molecules form a certain structure around dissolved molecules or ions, or in the case of applying an electrical field, because water molecules are dipoles (that is, they have a dipolar nature because of their structure and composition). This is science. But on the other hand, water molecules are in continual movement and, as a result, the bonds between them constantly switch from one molecule to another. The temporary bonds between particular water molecules last an infinitesimal time, of around 50 femtoseconds, which is 0.00000000000005 seconds.[27] Therefore "water-memory" is far too short to transmit the "information" of the initial raw substance. Only in a solid state (as ice) do these bonds become permanent and the water molecules form a stable structure. This problem gets even worse in the use of alcohol as a solvent, as was recommended by Hahnemann,[28] because alcohol molecules form much weaker bonds than those of water. And if an insoluble substance (such as metallic gold) is used, its mixing with lactose granules stretches imagination even further on how information could be passed on to successive "dilutions." In the end, even if there existed a structure "memorized" by the water molecules during successive dilutions, it would be lost when the final remedy was absorbed in lactose granules.[29]

As if Hahnemann had prefigured this tension between homeopathy and science, he discouraged from the very beginning the search for an explanation of how homeopathy works. He stated that "it is impossible only through the efforts of the intellect to recognize the spirit-like force

---

27. Cowan et al., "Ultrafast memory loss and energy redistribution," 199–202.

28. *Organon*, 270.

29. Bill Gray argues that stable structures formed by water molecules can be observed when applying an electric field (Gray, *Homeopathy*, 64). However, in producing homeopathic remedies there is no electromagnetic field present. Another argument is that ions determine the structuring of water molecules around them (Gray, *Homeopathy*, 63.). This is true, but a formation of such structures is no longer possible once the C_{12} potency is reached, for no molecule or ion is left to structure water molecules around it.

itself, which, hidden in the intimate essence of the remedies, gives them the power to change the way people feel and thereby to cure diseases."[30] In the preface to his other fundamental work, *The Chronic Diseases*, Hahnemann affirmed that he did not "venture to explain how the cure of diseases is effected," for it is not necessary. All that matters is the result, being healed.[31]

So it is time to assess homeopathy from a metaphysical perspective, starting with the way it defines human nature. For one who wants to reconcile homeopathy with Christianity, this is where we start to find disturbing facts.

8.5 THE VITAL FORCE

Like most forms of alternative medicine, homeopathy rejects a materialistic view of human nature. Hahnemann affirms that the life of the physical body is sustained by an immaterial substance:

> In the healthy human state, the spirit-like life force (autocracy) that enlivens the material organism as dynamis, governs without restriction and keeps all parts of the organism in admirable, harmonious, vital operation, as regards both feelings and functions, so that our indwelling, rational spirit can freely avail itself of this living, healthy instrument for the higher purposes of our existence.[32]

Let us notice some important aspects of this "life force" (also called "vital force"): it has an immaterial nature, it animates the physical body and upholds its well-being, and makes us capable of having a rational life. The vital force cannot regain its balance by itself, so we were given "that greatest gift of God, the reflective intellect and the unrestrained power of deliberation"[33] to help it recover. As we can see, the vital force and reason are in a close relationship. On the one hand, the vital force has an irrational

---

30. *Organon*, 20.
31. Hahnemann, *The Chronic Diseases*, 20.
32. *Organon*, 9. Concerning the "higher purposes of our existence" to which we should aspire, we must remember that deism grants total autonomy to reason in formulating the meaning of life, so everyone is free to formulate these "higher purposes" for oneself. Although Hahnemann mentioned God and providence (which led him to the discovery of homeopathy), we must remember he spoke as a deist, never as a committed Christian. I found no clue in his biography and letters that he ever expressed Christian beliefs.
33. *Organon*, "Introduction."

nature; is not guided by reason, but upholds the function of reason. On the other hand, only reason can find the proper remedies for healing the vital force and thus for regaining health.[34]

Illness is the result of the weakening of this immaterial component of our nature, in a similar way in which other forms of alternative medicine state it as a weakening of the etheric body. Hahnemann emphasizes that diseases "are not mechanical or chemical alterations of the material substance of the organism; they are not dependent on material disease matter. They are solely spirit-like, dynamic mistunements of life."[35] In other words, unlike in Western medicine, an illness does not have a material origin, such as microbes, viruses or mechanical blockages in our body, but is

> engendered by a spirit-like inimical potence that disturbs, as if by a kind of contagion, the spirit-like life principle that reigns, with its instinctual governance, in the entire organism. Like an evil spirit, it torments the life principle, forcing it to engender certain sufferings and disorders in the course of its life.[36]

Modern homeopaths affirm that such statements do not negate the role of pathogens, but should be understood as meaning that the true cause of disease is the weakening of the body due to the weakening of its vital force. This makes possible the attack of microbes and viruses. Another approach is that of Vithoulkas, who argues that an illness can be seen as an interaction between the vital force of the ill person and that of the microbes: "It is not the microbes or the virus or the bacteria, nor even their virulent

---

34. In Hahnemann's words, "The life force, that glorious power innate in the human being, was ordained to conduct life in the most perfect way *during its health*. The life force, which is equally present in all parts of the organism (in the sensible as well as the irritable fiber) is the untiring mainspring of all normal natural bodily functions. It was not at all created for the purpose of helping itself in diseases nor for exercising a medical art worthy of imitation" (*Organon*, "Introduction").

35. *Organon*, 31, footnote.

36. *Organon*, 148. Contrary to modern medicine, Hahnemann argued that infectious diseases such as smallpox or measles are not transmitted from one child to another through physical contact. In his words, "this contamination takes place invisibly (dynamically) at a distance, without something material having come (or having been able to come) into the affected child from the contagious one, just as there is no material transmission between the magnet and the steel needle. A solely specific, spirit-like impingement communicates smallpox or measles from one child to another nearby, just as a magnet communicates the magnetic property to a steel needle nearby" (*Organon*, 11, footnote).

poisons on the biochemical level that cause disease, but rather their intimate nature, their vital force, their very 'soul.'"[37]

Hahnemann does not provide a clear explanation of how the weakness of the vital force develops into a disease. He simply affirms that "the disease-tuned life force alone brings forth diseases,"[38] and that a clear understanding of how this happens is not possible:

> The medical-art practitioner can derive no benefit from probing into how and why the life force brings the organism to the manifestations of disease, that is, how it creates disease. This will remain eternally hidden from him. The Lord of life laid before his senses only what was necessary and fully sufficient for him to be aware of for curative purposes.[39]

Kent is more generous in explaining the mechanism of healing. He argues that the role of the homeopathic remedy is to strengthen the vital force by giving it the energy of a certain raw substance, which is released and potentized during succussion. In his view, not only are living beings kept alive by this mysterious vital force, but all substances have such an immaterial component (a "simple substance") that makes them what they are:

> The simple substance gives to everything its own type of life, gives it distinction, gives it identity whereby it differs, from all other things. The crystal of the earth has its own association, its own identity; it is endowed with a simple substance that will establish its identity from everything in the animal kingdom, everything in the mineral kingdom.[40]

This approach reminds us of how Aquinas defined things as being composed of matter and form. The "simple substance" of Kent, which provides the identity of a certain thing, is the equivalent of what Aquinas defined as "form." Once we grasp this similarity, we observe that by succussion the simple substance of a plant, animal or mineral is released. In Kent's words, "We also potentize our medicines in order to arrive at their simple substance; that is, at the nature and quality of the remedy itself."[41]

---

37. Vithoulkas, *Homeopathy: Medicine for the New Millennium*, 37.
38. *Organon*, 12.
39. *Organon*, 12, footnote.
40. Kent, *Lectures*, 79.
41. Kent, *Lectures*, 87.

This "simple substance" of the remedy is what heals the human vital force, not the raw substance in the lowest possible dose, as the second principle of homeopathy claims. This is why higher dilutions are stronger in effect, contrary to the logic of chemistry. Illness is overcome by the simple (immaterial) substance of the homeopathic remedy, which has been extracted through succussion. Only that immaterial essence can interact with one's immaterial vital force and heal it. Hahnemann expresses the same thought, although not with the same clarity, when he affirms:

> By means of this mechanical processing (. . .) a given medicinal substance which, in its crude state, is only matter (in some cases, unmedicinal matter) is subtilized and transformed by these higher and higher dynamizations to become a spirit-like medicinal power.[42]

As we can see, we are dealing here with a completely different logic from that of science. This is why a scientific explanation of how homeopathy works cannot be found. Its mechanism is metaphysical. Illness has a metaphysical cause, the weakening of the (immaterial) vital force, so healing must be done at the same metaphysical level.

For a Christian this should sound alarming, for our immaterial nature is the soul, and our soul cannot interact with nature's simple substances, for there is a fundamental difference between the nature of our soul and the "soul" of plants and animals. In the order of creation we are *not* of the same kind with them.

8.6 THE VITAL FORCE AND MESMERISM. HOMEOPATHY AS ENERGY TRANSFER

An interesting aspect that can cast more light on the nature of the vital force is Hahnemann's favorable attitude towards mesmerism, a practice highly esteemed during his lifetime. Franz Anton Mesmer (1734–1815) was a German physician who argued that every living being possesses an inner force called "animal magnetism," whose flow in the body determines the state of health or illness. Early in his practice Mesmer claimed to be able to cure deficiencies of this energy in ill people by applying magnets on their body. Later he claimed to be himself the source of healing energy and to be able to transfer it to his patients by making magnetic passes over the body, by

---

42. *Organon*, 270.

pressing certain zones, or by giving patients "magnetized water" to drink. His method was discredited in 1784, when King Louis the XVIth of France demanded an investigation of Mesmer's claims by the Faculty of Medicine of Paris, which proved that mesmerism can work only as a placebo.

But Hahnemann was very favorable to mesmerism, and called it "a wonderful, priceless gift of God, granted to humanity."[43] In his view, it was a way of healing the vital force of an ill person by a direct transfer of energy from the vital force of a healthy mesmerizer:

> A healthy mesmerist, gifted with this power, dynamically streams into another human being by means of touch or even without it—indeed even at some distance. It does so through the powerful will of a well-intentioned individual. The mesmerist's life force dynamically streams into another human being just as one of the poles of a powerful magnet dynamically streams into a rod of raw steel.[44]

This mechanism of energy transfer reminds us of Reiki healing. While in Reiki the healer channels *Chi* from the Universal Source to the one who needs it, in mesmerism this "life force" is transferred from the mesmerizer to the patient without mentioning a Universal Source. As Hahnemann argues, mesmerism

> replaces the life force lacking here and there in the patient's organism and in part, it drains off, decreases and more equally distributes the life force that has accumulated all-too-much in other places, thereby arousing and maintaining unnamable nervous sufferings. In general, it extinguishes the morbid mistunement of the patient's life principle, replacing it with the mesmerist's normal tunement which is powerfully impinging upon the patient.[45]

The mesmerizer is thus seen as possessing a strong vital force that can be directed to heal the weak vital force of the patient. This art of healing seems to be a quick alternative to traditional homeopathic practice, skipping the long interview and the effort of finding the right remedy in a homeopathic repertory. It is a simple energy transfer, and thus brings homeopathy in line with other energy-based techniques such as Reiki and acupuncture.

43. *Organon*, 288.
44. *Organon*, 288.
45. *Organon*, 288.

In the *Organon*, Hahnemann recommends rapid energy passes "by means of a very rapid movement of the flat out-stretched right hand, held parallel to and about an inch from the body, going from the top of the head down over the tips of the toes."[46] At the first congress of the Homeopathic Society (Leipzig, 1830), he recommended the use of mesmerism in case of a severe psora eruption, as an alternative to using homeopathic remedies. The prescribed procedure was that "a healthy person applies the thumb or the finger-tips tightly pressed together very close to the diseased part for a minute or two, each day, by which means new vitality would be awakened and supported in this part."[47] As Hahnemann wrote in a letter, in a situation where homeopathic remedies did not work because of allopathic medication abuse, a little girl was cured by her father, at Hahnemann's suggestion, "with the help of a few slow mesmeric passes."[48]

Having had such an enthusiastic attitude towards mesmerism, Hahnemann may have been open to what exists today as Reiki, and may have endorsed it. But if homeopathy is a form of energy transfer in which the role of the mesmerizer is played by the homeopathic remedies, we are facing the same problems for Christians that we found in other related forms of energy transfer. A contemporary advocate of this energy-related view of the vital force is the British homeopath Peter Chappell. He argues that, according to quantum physics, "we are a vibrational body of energy and that the physical reality we see and feel is only a construct of our brain."[49] The vital force organizes this "vibrational body of energy," and "disease occurs when there is a conflict between desired vitalizing action and actual effect owing to dynamic energy blockages."[50]

46. *Organon*, 289.

47. Haehl, *Samuel Hahnemann*, 267.

48. Haehl, *Samuel Hahnemann*, 291.

49. Chappell, *Emotional Healing*, 93. There are at least two other followers of this line of thought. See: Gina Tyler, *Homeopathy and Radiaesthesia*, online, and the Homeopathy Plus website, *The Vital Force*. Another confirmation that homeopathy could be seen as a kind of energy-transfer therapy comes from Morant, the master of acupuncture we followed in chapter 6. Referring to the nature of the vital force as defined by Hahnemann in the ninth aphorism of the *Organon*, he argues that Chinese philosophy has known "for more than four thousand years of the existence of this force" (Morant, *Chinese Acupuncture*, 185). While acupuncture balances *Chi* with the help of needles, homeopathy feeds it with its remedies. According to Morant, the imbalance of vital energy that Hahnemann sees as the cause of illness "is exactly this idea which is at the basis of the science of energy (acupuncture)" (Morant, *Chinese Acupuncture*, 293).

50. Chappell, *Emotional Healing*, 93.

Homeopathy

Chappell goes much deeper into speculating about the nature of the vital force and calls it "our connection to God."[51] However, this is not just an attempt to explain in homeopathic terms how we relate to God, as Christians may think. As Chappell argues, the vital force *is* part of *one* ultimate reality that includes God and us:

> I consider that our vitalizing force is our connection to God, we are God, or if you like, the energy of the ultimate intelligence of the universe that is all of every part of us.[52]

As we can see, from an energy-related view of human nature, Chappell has reached a perspective that represents it as divine. Failing to realize it and to listen to the demands of "our inner core" leads to getting physically sick. He affirms:

> This Godlike part of us, at the very core of us, we experience as a sense of Beingness, and this is what stands up, and when it/we withdraws, our body falls over. If we follow the dictates of our inner core Beingness, we are well, and when we systematically don't, we get sick. This sickness is a physicalized form of communication from our inner God to our outer personality, since the inner route is not being listened to.[53]

If we follow this energy-related view of human nature, we face similar issues with those mentioned in previous chapters. As such we can no longer be persons in relationship with God and neighbors, but grains of divine energy that need balancing by the use of homeopathic remedies. Christian homeopaths will, obviously, reject this view. But for them, the next section should pose problems that are no less worrying.

8.7 THE VITAL FORCE AND THE SOUL

The real difficulty that homeopathy should pose for Christians concerns the relationship between the meaning it ascribes to the vital force and the Christian meaning of the soul. In order to explore this topic we need to read carefully Kent's *Lectures on Homeopathic Philosophy*. He argues that human nature has three components: the material body, the immaterial vital force ("the vice-regent of the soul"), and another immaterial component called

---

51. Chappell, *Emotional Healing*, 94.
52. Chappell, *Emotional Healing*, 94.
53. Chappell, *Emotional Healing*, 94.

the interior man, or "the soul," which is composed of will and understanding.[54] Let us explore the relationship between these three components.

In the ninth aphorism of the *Organon* Hahnemann defines the vital force as sustaining both the life of the body and the action of reason. Following Hahnemann, Kent reaffirms the symbiotic relationship that exists between the vital force and the soul, arguing that the vital force "keeps the operation of mind and will in order,"[55] and that it cannot heal itself, so it needs the action of reason to pick the right remedies. Therefore, according to Hahnemann and Kent, the pillars of homeopathy, the vital force cannot be the equivalent of an etheric body, as found in other forms of alternative medicine. An etheric body is a link between higher spiritual bodies and the physical body, by no means one that sustains the higher spiritual bodies as the vital force does for the soul according to homeopathy.

As already mentioned in section 5 of this chapter, if we try to find the equivalent of the vital force in Christian teaching, we can identify it as the soul. Here is a statement on the relationship between the soul and the body that could easily be attributed to a Christian theologian familiar with the thought of Aquinas:

> The soul adapts the human body to all its purposes, the higher purposes of its being. The simple substance when it exists in the living human body keeps that body animated, keeps it moving, perfects its uses, superintends all parts and at the same time keeps the operation of mind and will in order. (. . .) in its absence there is death and destruction.[56]

However, this is not part of a Christian treatise of theology, but Kent's view of human nature, in which we find the operations of the vegetative, the locomotion, the appetitive and the intellectual powers of the soul. In a Christian reading, what Hahnemann and Kent call the vital force is not a second immaterial substance, besides the soul, but the lower powers of the soul itself. In the *Summa Theologiae* (I,78,1) Aquinas argues that the soul has five powers: vegetative, sensitive, appetitive, locomotion, and intellectual. He emphasizes that *all* these powers belong to the same soul, so they are not distinct entities in human nature, or different spiritual bodies, as we have seen in some forms of alternative medicine. Therefore what in homeopathy is the soul *and* the vital force, according to Christian theology

54. Kent, *Lectures*, 45. "Understanding" is used as a synonym for reason.
55. Kent, *Lectures*, 83.
56. Kent, *Lectures*, 83.

is simply *the soul* with its five powers. They cannot be separated into two substances or two spiritual bodies. They constitute a single soul, and thus the vital force can only be seen as a *part* of the soul.[57] Since homeopathy heals the vital force with the energy of its remedies, and this vital force can only be part of the soul, what homeopathy really attempts to heal with its remedies is *the soul*. And here we face a serious contradiction between homeopathy and the Christian view of human nature, for the soul can be cured only by the grace of God.

Aquinas indicates there is a similarity between a disease, as an illness of the body, and sin, as an illness of the soul: "We need to consider that sin consists of a disorder of the soul, just as physical disease consists of disorder of the body. And so sin is a disease of the soul, as it were, and pardon for sin is what healing is for disease."[58] This "pardon for sin," as healing for the soul, can only be effected by God, the Person against whom one has sinned, and by no means by a homeopathic remedy. The healing grace of God cannot be replaced by homeopathic remedies. The human soul is a special creation of God, with a different status from the life of animals and plants, and with a different destiny. The human soul is meant for eternal life, and thus can be healed only by its Creator through supernatural means, in an existing personal relationship with him. No immaterial essence extracted from plants, animals or minerals can cure it. This is the main problem that homeopathy should pose for Christians and convince them to reconsider its nature and "miraculous" benefits.

8.8 MIASMS AND ORIGINAL SIN

Another theological issue for Christians arises from the meaning of the miasm called psora. Kent defines it in terms which point to a derangement or infirmity of human nature much deeper than biological weakness. In his words, psora is "the primitive or primary disorder of the human race, (. . .) a disordered state of the internal economy of the human race."[59] It manifests

---

57. The Canadian homeopath Andrea Hauser affirms that the vital force is a component of human nature that enters at conception and leaves the body at death in a similar way to the Christian view of the soul: "The vital force is the animate force that enters the body at the time of conception, guides all life function, and leaves the body in death. It keeps each individual in tune & integrates the whole" (Hauser, *What is Homeopathic Medicine?*, online).

58. Aquinas, *On Evil*, VII,1, 269.

59. Kent, *Lectures*, 146.

itself as a moral weakness, and only due to this primarily moral disorder does one become prone to physical diseases:

> The state of the human mind and the state of the human body, is a state of susceptibility to disease from willing evils, from thinking that which is false and making life one continuous heredity of false things, and so this form of disease, Psora, is but an outward manifestation of that which is prior in man.[60]

A Christian could easily recognize here an analogy with what is called the doctrine of original sin. This analogy seems justified since the psoric condition can be traced back to the origin of the human race. Kent affirms: "If the human race had remained in a state of perfect order, psora could not have existed. (. . .) it goes to the very primitive wrong of the human race, the very first sickness of the human race, that is the spiritual sickness."[61]

The Indian homeopath N. Ghatak follows on the same lines. He argues that the origin of psora is in a defective way of thinking, which started when human beings made the first bad decisions consciously and willingly.[62] Psora is an inherited mental disorder that is gradually "reflected in the physical body."[63] It started "as soon as he (man) exercised the power of free will, with which he was endowed, and willed against the laws of God,"[64] and became an "internal itching of the mind."[65] How could we better translate to a Christian this predisposition to negative thinking, which is "transmitted from generation to generation,"[66] than the doctrine of original sin, formulated in homeopathic terms?

---

60. Kent, *Lectures*, 156.

61. Kent, *Lectures*, 146. He also says that "the children inherit it from their parents and carry it on and continue it" (Kent, *Lectures*, 158.).

62. Banerjee, *Chronic Disease*, 6–7. This is a translation of N. Ghatak's original Bengali into English.

63. Banerjee, *Chronic Disease*, 6.

64. Banerjee, *Chronic Disease*, 69. A longer quote is necessary here: "Man was not born ill. We cannot conceive that God who is goodness and greatness only, could have made man otherwise than good and great. The good, healthy man was living out his life in purity and health. God gave man goodness, but he gave man also the power to be bad. Man was good, and God, his Creator desired him to be good, but God gave him the power of free will and free action. (. . .) But as soon as he exercised the power of free will, with which he was endowed, and willed against the laws of God, the trouble began" (Banerjee, *Chronic Disease*, 69).

65. Banerjee, *Chronic Disease*, 6–7.

66. Banerjee, *Chronic Disease*, 8.

Kent is right in saying that our "internal order" is deeply affected and this inherited spiritual condition makes us "thinking evils and willing falses."[67] This is the state of sin, which is indeed our fundamental problem. It is both a personal problem in daily life, for we sin as individuals by our thoughts, words, works and omissions, and a state we inherit as representatives of the human race, called original sin. The Catholic Catechism teaches:

> Adam and Eve transmitted to their descendants human nature wounded by their own first sin and hence deprived of original holiness and justice; this deprivation is called "original sin." As a result of original sin, human nature is weakened in its powers, subject to ignorance, suffering and the domination of death, and inclined to sin (this inclination is called 'concupiscence').[68]

However, this state cannot be healed with energy-impregnated sugar globules, for our soul is not a substance similar to other substances in the mineral, plant or animal world, that it may interact with the energy of these remedies. As stated in the previous section, our soul can be healed only by the grace of God, for it was created by him and subsists on his grace alone. Homeopaths like Kent and Ghatak have correctly identified a deep seated problem in human nature, but failed to acknowledge its proper remedy.

8.9 A PERSONAL ENCOUNTER WITH HOMEOPATHY

Twenty-six years ago, I was a patient of a homeopath doctor. I did not know anything at that time about homeopathy. A (Christian) friend told me that homeopathy works, and that he experienced in himself its healing power. So I went to the (Christian) homeopathic doctor he recommended. There were two strange things that made me question the nature of this healing art. The first was the interview, in which was established my general character and miasm. I was asked questions completely unrelated to medicine. How is my sleep, what are my dreams like, at what time do I wake up at night, what are my fears, etc. The other element was the chemistry of homeopathic remedies. As I was a chemistry teacher at that time, I wondered how these remedies could work since there was no molecule of active substance left in the prescribed remedy, except the "energy" it had acquired during potentization. The first remedy I was supposed to take was

---

67. Kent, *Lectures*, 159.
68. CCC 417–18.

Nux Vomica.[69] Before taking it, as a precautionary measure, I prayed that God would protect me from any harmful, unseen, non-physical "forces" that might be associated with this weird "medicine."

I had been warned that my body would react strongly to the given remedy and manifest symptoms such as vomiting, nausea and intestinal cramping, which I had to interpret as the elimination of toxins accumulated over many years of allopathic medication. After that initial state of feeling worse, everything would eventually improve. I did not suffer from any grave illness, but like most people, I had the miasm called psora. To my surprise, I had absolutely no reaction to *Nux Vomica* or to the other remedies, which I took one at a time, as prescribed, over a period of two months. The only reaction was my frustration of not being allowed to drink coffee, black tea or Coca-Cola, which are said to poison the body. A very interesting aspect is that my friend, who recommended this homeopathic doctor, had also started with *Nux Vomica*, but in his case, the warnings came true and he went through a nasty period of "purgation" with all its foretold manifestations.

What happened in my case? Did my lack of trust in the remedies cancel their effect? Did it cancel a placebo effect? Did the remedies work without any symptoms? Or was I guarded against being affected by a mysterious force? It was much later that I learned about the spiritual teachings of homeopathy that I have shared in this chapter. The mysterious nature of the vital force, its correspondence to the soul and the aim of homeopathy to cure the vital force, and thus the soul, should raise a red flag for a Christian. The healing of the soul is possible only as God has revealed it, by the grace that flows from him.[70] Any Christian should be aware of this before trying out homeopathy.

8.10 ADDENDUM. THE BACH FLORAL REMEDIES

A form of alternative medicine related to homeopathy, at least through its founder, is the one developed by the English physician Edward Bach (1886–1936). Although it is usually taken as a form of phytotherapy, as we discover its spiritual teachings it becomes obvious that Bach floral

---

69. This is a remedy prepared from the fruit of the poison nut tree (or strychnine tree), known for its high concentration of strychnine.

70. Catholic and Eastern Orthodox Christians would add here: by the grace that flows from God *through the sacraments.*

remedies work on spiritual grounds which are blatantly incompatible with Christianity.

Bach studied medicine at Birmingham and London (1906–1912), and began his MD career in 1913. He specialized in immunology and bacteriology, and then worked as a researcher at the Homeopathic hospital in London. At the age of 43 he quit and dedicated himself to establishing a new healing method that would be completely natural. In 1935, one year before his death, he declared this project accomplished by finding the 38 floral remedies that bear his name.

There are two methods by which Bach remedies are prepared. The first, called the *Sun Method*, uses the flowers of certain plants. They are put in a bowl of spring water and left in direct sunlight for three hours, on the assumption that solar radiation transfers the pure energy of the flowers into water. Then the flowers are discarded, one adds the same amount of brandy as that of the remaining water, and the floral tincture is ready. This method produces 20 of the 38 Bach floral remedies. The other 18 are obtained by the *Boiling Method*. Small branches that have blossomed are boiled for half an hour, and then the procedure continues as the *Sun Method*. A few drops of the right tincture are added to a glass of water and sipped over the day until the patient feels better. If one has a more serious illness several remedies at a time need to be taken.

Bach presented his method as superior to homeopathy. He admired Hahnemann, but asked his followers to take the next step in the art of healing and adopt his method. Instead of producing remedies out of toxic raw substances, as in classic homeopathy, he argued it was time to use completely natural and non-toxic sources.[71] He thought that if Hahnemann had continued his activity "he would have progressed along these lines. We are merely advancing his work, and carrying it to the next natural stage."[72]

According to Bach, disease "is the natural consequence of disharmony between our bodies and our Souls."[73] The soul, in Bach's view, is an immaterial substance of divine origin, "a Vital and Immortal Principle."[74] However, this is not the Christian view of the soul, but rather corresponds closely to the Hindu self (*atman*). In a similar way to other forms of alternative medicine, the noblest part of our nature, the soul, is "a Spark of

---

71. Bach, *Ye suffer from Yourselves*, 8.
72. Bach, *Ye suffer from Yourselves*, 9.
73. Bach, *Ye suffer from Yourselves*, 7.
74. Bach, *The Wallingford Lectures*, 25.

the Divine."⁷⁵ Therefore the above definition of disease can be rephrased as a "disharmony between yourself and the Divinity within you,"⁷⁶ which should already serve as a warning about this therapy.

The element that generates the conflict between the "spiritual self" and the body is not sin in a Christian sense, but ignorance in knowing our true nature. Once spiritual ignorance is healed, the two components of our nature live in harmony. In Bach's words, "the amount of peace, of happiness, of joy, of health and of well-being that comes into our lives depends also on the amount of which the Divine Spark can enter and illuminate our existence."⁷⁷ All we need for our well-being can be found in the 38 flower remedies, both to heal and to "bring us nearer to the Divinity within."⁷⁸ As in other forms of alternative medicine such as Ayurveda or Reiki, real healing is produced by the "increase of the Divinity within."⁷⁹ Therefore, an illness is ultimately a means of spiritual evolution, a message that our "divine" soul sends "to point out to us our faults, to prevent our making greater errors, to hinder us from doing more harm, and to bring us back to that path of Truth and Light from which we should never have strayed."⁸⁰ As we can see, the esoteric side of healing with Bach's floral remedies is much easier to identify than in homeopathy. Remedies are given not only to regain health, but also as means of spiritual growth towards knowing our alleged divine nature.

The ultimate purpose of our existence is to "develop our individuality that we may obtain complete freedom to serve the Divinity within ourselves, and that Divinity alone."⁸¹ No grace or external help is needed for us to reach perfection, for we have all resources in our divine self. Bach affirms:

> We, as children of the Creator, have within us all perfection, and
> we come into this world merely that we may realise our Divinity;

75. Bach, *The Wallingford Lectures*, 25.
76. Bach, *Ye suffer from Yourselves*, 11.
77. Bach, *The Wallingford Lectures*, 25–26.
78. Bach, *The Wallingford Lectures*, 26.
79. Bach, *The Wallingford Lectures*, 26.
80. Bach, *Ye suffer from Yourselves*, 10. For instance, problems in the hand indicates "failure or wrong in action: the foot, failure to assist others: the brain, lack of control: the heart, deficiency or excess, or wrong doing in the aspect of love: the eye, failure to see aright and comprehend the truth when placed before you" (*Ye suffer from Yourselves*, 11–12).
81. Bach, *Ye suffer from Yourselves*, 23.

so that all tests and all experiences will leave us untouched, for through that Divine Power all things are possible to us.[82]

The meaning of sin is summed up in one principle, "that of not obeying the dictates of our own Divinity. That is the sin against God and our neighbour."[83] Therefore we should not follow "wishes and desires of other people so often implanted in our minds, or of conscience, which is another word for the same thing."[84] Anything we have been taught so far as traditional (Christian) wisdom is a way by which the world "wishes to enslave us."[85] Bach urges his followers to live in total autonomy from (traditional) external influences and to know the truth by their own efforts.[86] One is himself or herself the measure of all things, and sin is precisely the refusal of this self-sufficiency.

The contradiction that Bach's philosophy poses to Christianity cannot be clearer. Contrary to his claims, we have no infallible inner voice. Our conscience must be formed by traditional Christian teaching and be illuminated by grace, and we cannot reach perfection unassisted by grace and the fellowship of the Christian community.

Bach makes astonishing claims of his remedies not only for Christians, but for practitioners of other forms of alternative medicine as well. Not only do these remedies heal physical illnesses, but they can also be taken as an instant fix for spiritual ignorance and any weakness of the soul. Consider the following examples: Aspen (the remedy produced from the trembling aspen) is good for "fear, by day and night for known reason" such as darkness, death, and disaster,[87] while Mimulus treats "fear of death, accidents, poverty, people and animals." Those who lack hope have no need of faith, but need to take Gorse (made of wild barley); and the egocentric who does not care about anyone can be healed with Heather (black grass). Hate, envy, and greed are not sins, but mere weaknesses which can be treated with Holly, and those who lack patience can take Impatiens. The sense of

---

82. Bach, *Free Thyself*, 25.
83. Bach, *Free Thyself*, 15.
84. Bach, *Free Thyself*, 15.
85. Bach, *Free Thyself*, 15–16.
86. This self-sufficiency means rejecting all "outside influences" (*Free Thyself*, 15), but obviously not those stated by Bach.
87. This is an example of the rationale that stands behind choosing his remedies. Since fear is manifested by trembling, the remedy for it must be produced from a plant that mimics trembling.

guilt, the rebuke of conscience when one has done evil, is healed with Pine; and the discouraged and depressed do not need to pray, but take Gentian. Cherry Plum heals "desperation, fear of suicide, insanity or murderous impulses," while Crab Apple heals "feelings of despair, uncleanness, those who feel mentally and physically unclean."[88]

We can easily see how antagonistic the underlying philosophy of this therapy is to Christianity. Since any spiritual weakness and any rebuke of our conscience for a sin can be solved with a certain remedy, repentance is done away with. Instead of struggling with temptations and weaknesses by the power of grace, we can get a quick fix by a few drops of these 38 miraculous Bach floral remedies. This is not just an overstatement of the power of natural remedies, but a profoundly anti-Christian teaching on human nature.

---

88. All these prescriptions are found in Master et al., *Bach Flower Remedies*, 9–39.

9

Alternative Medicine and the Christian View of Health and Healing

THERE ARE MANY OTHER forms of alternative medicine that I have not addressed in this book.[1] You can probably name several others that you have heard of or even used for healing. Instead of an exhaustive (and exhausting) presentation of many forms, I have rather intended this book as a "toolkit" for enabling you to evaluate any form of alternative medicine and to judge for yourself to what extent it is compatible with Christian faith. Let us remember the guiding thoughts mentioned at the end of the first chapter. On the one hand, Catholic teaching is that:

> Being in the image of God the human individual possesses the dignity of a person, who is not just something, but someone. He is capable of self-knowledge, of self-possession, and of freely giving himself and entering into communion with other persons. And he is called by grace to a covenant with his Creator, to offer him a response of faith and love that no other creature can give in his stead.[2]

On the other hand, Karl Barth emphasized from a Protestant perspective that:

> Just as man is distinguished from the rest of the created world by the fact that, as the likeness and promise of the divine covenant

---

1. I look forward to getting your feedback for an improved edition. You can send comments and suggestions on this email address: ernestmariusoo@yahoo.com. Please make your suggestions as clear and objective as possible.

2. CCC 357.

> of grace, he is called to responsibility before God, so his special constitution corresponding to this calling is determined by the fact that he owes it to the God who is the Lord of this covenant of grace.[3]

Since all forms of alternative medicine that we have met in this book have a "spiritual" side, which of them allows us to give God "a response of faith and love" or be responsible partners in "a covenant of grace"? Yoga teaches us to follow the principles and goal of Hinduism, that of reaching union with an impersonal ultimate reality. To achieve perfection as a person in the afterlife is absurd, and so is the goal of Christianity. Ayurveda presents itself as a phytotherapy and a guide for a balanced lifestyle, but behind this veil lies a subtle invitation to experience Hindu philosophy and meditation. Anthroposophical medicine follows the teachings of its founder, and thus invites us to develop our divine soul and enter into communion with Luciferic spirits. Acupuncture and reflexology teach us that we are a complex energy system that must remain in harmony with universal energy. The relation that is established between us and ultimate reality is summed up as a flow of *Chi* energy, from a Source to a receiver. There is no space left in this balancing of energies for personal communion and love. In Reiki we can benefit from the help of spirits called "angels" or "deities." They teach us about karma, reincarnation, and our divine nature. In homeopathy we let our soul be healed with homeopathic remedies instead of God's grace. Bach floral remedies silence any rebuke of conscience with herbal extracts. In short, this is the spiritual side of alternative medicine. Does it encourage us to love God? What is God according to these spiritual teachings? Can we follow these views and grow in faith? What is faith according to them? And what is the ultimate fulfillment of the human being according to these spiritual views? Answer these questions and check the right answers in your particular Christian tradition. Then draw your own conclusions.

We often hear that alternative medicine is superior to classical medicine, for it treats us holistically, that is, as a whole, both the physical body and the immaterial part of our nature. Although such an approach seems desirable, it is precisely this aspect that opens the door to spiritual views incompatible with Christianity. While affirming that the whole person needs to be cured, many forms of alternative medicine define the "immaterial" part of our nature in ways that would supersede Christian faith. The origin

---

3. Barth, *Church Dogmatics*, III,2, 347.

of physical illness is found in *that* immaterial part, as the manifestation of an energy imbalance. In the chapter on homeopathy I argued that the soul cannot be healed with the energy contained in sugar globules, but only with the grace of God, because the soul is made by him and has a special nature, unlike anything else in creation. This principle can be applied to all other forms of alternative medicine that claim to heal a spiritual body or rebalance *Chi* or *prana* energy. The soul is not an "energy" and cannot be healed by such means, for it is a special creation of God at the moment of conception. Only if God creates the soul able to "offer a response of faith and love" and thus make us responsible partners in "a covenant of grace" can faith and love have any meaning. A spiritual essence, an energy, the universe, or any other such impersonal ultimate reality that would "balance" our own energy, cannot provide the ground for making human nature capable of love, or to make sense of an everlasting relationship of love.

To summarize the essence of this book, there are a few principles we can follow to assess the spiritual side of any form of alternative medicine. Any claim to one or more of the following is a call to experience a spirituality alien to Christianity. Here are the claims that should raise red flags:

- Human nature has a divine component, or an essence of the same nature as the divine, of which we must become aware;
- Everything that exists is part of a single spiritual essence;
- We must keep the right balance with a universal energy;
- We are a miniature of the universe, and we can find its principles and mechanism inside ourselves;
- We have inside us all the resources to reach perfection, and need only initiation;
- There are hidden powers we can tap, or we can benefit from the help of "spirits" or "deities."

Being healed by a form of alternative medicine which works on such assumptions will stimulate the desire to know more of that spirituality and can eventually lead to one's estrangement, and ultimately to the loss of faith, which would be the greatest loss one can imagine.

Now let us pause for a moment from thinking about the spiritual dimension of alternative medicine and ponder whether a similar twist of beliefs can be induced by classic Western medicine. Since it speaks nothing of a spiritual side of our nature, could it lead one to embrace a naturalist view of the world, according to which nature and its laws are all there is? In other words, can classic medicine lead to atheism? Not necessarily. One that follows naturalism and rejects faith is simply filling the emptiness of the soul with a materialistic philosophy. Western medicine does not work on a spiritual basis. As Christians we believe that it is God who gives us the necessary wisdom to discover the mechanisms that rule our physical body, and therefore a Christian can give all credit for his or her healing to God, not to science itself. To replace God with science (even medical science) means following a philosophy called scientism, which assumes that everything must be explained scientifically, and nothing can exist outside the realm of science. But following this philosophy is not a requirement of Western medicine, and this is the reason why many medical doctors call themselves Christians.

Western medicine, despite its materialist orientation, does not uphold a working principle that could take the place of Christian faith. It is precisely because it does *not* speak of energies that feed our soul, and because it does not speak at all about the soul, that it leaves room for Christian faith to fill this gap. As we have seen in chapter 1, Christianity can easily correct the materialistic perspective on human nature. A medical doctor can be a Christian without contradicting the principles of modern medicine, nor his or her faith, while a healer of most forms of alternative medicine cannot accommodate Christianity within the esoteric teachings of these techniques. Hence, the holistic approach of alternative medicine can be a trap for a Christian, not an advantage over classical medicine.

Christianity affirms healing both through the means of medical science and through supernatural means. However, its supernatural means for healing are not a kind of magic which works regardless of the circumstances and faith of the person concerned. For instance, in the Catholic and Eastern Orthodox traditions there is a special sacrament dedicated to healing, called the Anointing of the Sick. According to the Catholic Catechism, its purpose is to confer "a special grace on the Christian experiencing the difficulties inherent in the condition of grave illness or old age."[4] One of the fruits of this sacrament is "the restoration of health, *if* it is conducive to the salvation of (the person's) soul."[5]

Medical and supernatural means for restoring health are not mutually exclusive, and Christianity has a long history of providing medical help

---

4. CCC 1527.

5. CCC 1532, emphasis mine.

from its very beginning. Not to seek health when we get ill would be irresponsible and absurd, for our family and society need us. But to seek health through means that compromise our faith and salvation is quite another story. We have to keep in mind that health is not an end in itself, but a means for fulfilling the higher purpose of our life, that of offering God "a response of faith and love" and becoming a responsible partner in "a covenant of grace." Just as wealth, beauty, and fame are passing away no matter how much we cling to them, health will eventually also pass away, for we are all mortal. Despite all advances in medical science, and despite the skills of all masters of alternative medicine, the mortality rate is still 100 percent. Therefore, health should not become an idol, our reason for living, or the means that enables a hedonistic lifestyle.

Interestingly enough, the masters of alternative medicine also urge us to seek the deeper meaning of life, that which lies beyond the health of the physical body. For example, the Reiki master Arjava Petter invites us to ask ourselves "Who Am I?," and argues that when "that question is answered, all suffering comes to an end."[6] His answer, however, as we have seen in the chapter on Reiki, is that our nature is defined by our "divine core," also called "the true, divine self," or "the little flame of spiritual consciousness." To the same question Deepak Chopra, the master of Ayurveda, gives a similar answer: "I am pure consciousness, pure potentiality, a field of all possibilities."[7] Thus Petter, Chopra and many other masters of alternative medicine invite us to discover a so-called divine nature hidden in the depths of our being. For a Christian such views are unacceptable, because we do not have a divine nature. According to Christian teaching, we are God's creatures and will never surpass a creaturely condition.

Unlike the religious views of most forms of alternative medicine, Christianity teaches that human beings do not find their meaning through attaining harmony with a universal energy such as *Chi*, *Ki* or *Prana*. We find our meaning in relationship with God, our Creator, by opening ourselves towards him in faith and love. This is the foundation of a Christian's perspective on life and health, and also the reason why a disease can serve as a warning against a superficial, self-centered, and ignorant way of life. Our call is to holiness, to be set apart from anything that diverts us from loving God and our neighbors, to strive for moral perfection and the perfect service of God.

6. Lübeck et al., *The Spirit of Reiki*, 189.
7. Chopra, *Power, Freedom and Grace*, 62.

We will achieve perfect health only when we get a perfect resurrected body in the life to come. Meanwhile our target is holiness. For a Christian there is no direct correlation between personal holiness and the health of the body. Since the source of life is God, not an energy that we can control or balance, to be ill is not necessarily a sign of spiritual imperfection. Consider the lives of the saints. Can you name *one* that was spared of suffering? All went through hardships. Many are martyrs for the faith. Many died in their youth from grave illnesses. Consider just three: Therese of Lisieux, Bernadette, and Faustina. They died of tuberculosis, at the ages of 24, 35, and 33. Read their biographies and wonder at what great saints God made of them through suffering.

If we face a serious illness and have exhausted all admissible means to find healing, we must accept suffering and be convinced that it will fulfill the will of God in our life. He allows illnesses to draw our attention to the higher purpose of life, that of reaching holiness. Sometimes he does not heal us at all, and then we need to be capable of declaring, as did the apostle Paul:

> I have competed well; I have finished the race; I have kept the faith. From now on the crown of righteousness awaits me, which the Lord, the just judge, will award to me on that day, and not only to me, but to all who have longed for his appearance (2 Tim 4,7–8).

Let the sufferings that God allows in our lives not harden our heart, but soften our soul and lead us to holiness, that we might receive that crown of righteousness!

Bibliography

Aquinas, Thomas. *On Evil.* Oxford: Oxford University Press, 2003.
———. *Questions on the Soul.* Milwaukee: Marquette University Press, 1984.
———. *Summa Theologiae,* vol. I, translators: Fathers of the English Dominican Province, London: Burns Oates & Washbourne, 1920.
Bach, Edward. *Free Thyself.* Brightwell-cum-Sotwell (UK): The Bach Centre, 2014.
———. *The Wallingford Lectures.* Brightwell-cum-Sotwell (UK): The Bach Centre, 2014.
———. *Ye suffer from Yourselves.* Brightwell-cum-Sotwell (UK): The Bach Centre, 2015.
Banerjee, P.N. *Chronic Disease – Its Cause and Cure.* New Delhi: B. Jain Publishers, 1986.
Barth, Karl. *Church Dogmatics,* III,2, Edinburgh: T. & T. Clark, 1960.
———. *Dogmatics in Outline,* New York: Harper & Brothers, 1959.
Boericke, William. *Pocket Manual of Homeopathic Materia Medica.* New York: Boericke & Runyon, 1906 (online source: www.homeoint.org/books/boericmm/n/nat-m.htm, retrieved December 13, 2019).
Bott, Victor. *Anthroposophische Medizin: Band II. Planeten und Metalle* [*Anthroposophical Medicine, vol. II, Planets and Metals*]. Heidelberg: Haug, 1987.
Bradford, Thomas Lindsley. *The Life and Letters of Dr. Samuel Hahnemann.* Philadelphia: Boericke & Tafee, 1895.
Chappell, Peter. *Emotional Healing with Homeopathy: Treating the Effects of Trauma.* Berkeley: North Atlantic, 2003.
Chopra, Deepak. *Boundless Energy: The Complete Mind/Body Program for Overcoming Chronic Fatigue.* New York: Three Rivers, 1995.
———. *How to Know God: The Soul's Journey into the Mystery of Mysteries* (large print). New York: Random House, 2000.
———. "'I Am That,' A Secret Teaching Comes Home for All of Us," online source: www.chopra.com/ccl/i-am-that-a-secret-teaching-comes-home-for-all-of-us, (retrieved December 10, 2019).
———. *Perfect Health* (updated edition). New York: Three Rivers, 2000.
———. *Perfect Health: The Complete Mind/Body Guide.* Toronto: Bantam Books, 1990.
———. *Power, Freedom and Grace: Living from the Source of Lasting Happiness.* San Rafael, CA: Amber-Allen, 2006.
———. *Reinventing the Body, Resurrecting the Soul.* New York: Three Rivers, 2010.
Core, Christine. *Angelic Reiki: "The Healing for Our Time," Archangel Metatron.* Bloomington, IN: Balboa, 2011.
Cosway-Hayes, Joan. *Reflexology for Every Body.* Calgary: Footloose, 1996.

Bibliography

Cowan, M. L. et al., "Ultrafast memory loss and energy redistribution in the hydrogen bond network of liquid H2O," *Nature*, 434 (2005): 199–202.

Dasgupta, Surendranath. *A History of Indian Philosophy*, vol. I-II. Delhi: Motilal Banarsidass, 1975.

Eliade, Mircea. *A History of Religious Ideas*, vol. I-II. Chicago: University of Chicago Press, 1978.

———. *Yoga: Immortality and Freedom*. New York: Routledge & Kegan Paul, 1958.

Eliade, Mircea, and Couliano, Ioan P. *The Eliade Guide to World Religions*. New York: HarperCollins, 1991.

Gary Stewart, et al. *Basic Questions on Alternative Medicine*. Grand Rapids: Kregel, 1998.

Goldacre, Ben. *Bad Science*. London: Fourth Estate, 2008.

Gray, Bill. *Homeopathy. Science or Myth?* Berkeley: North Atlantic, 2000.

Guillaume, Madeleine J., Tymowski, Jean-Claude, Fiévet-Izard, Madeleine. *L'acupuncture*. Paris: Presses Universitaires de France, 2010.

Haehl, Richard. *Samuel Hahnemann, His Life and Work*. London: Homeopathic Publishing Company, 1922.

Hahnemann, Samuel. *Organon of the Medical Art*. Palo Alto, CA: Birdcage, 1996.

———. *The Chronic Diseases, Their Peculiar Nature and their Homeopathic Cure*. Philadelphia: Boericke & Tafel, 1896 (onnline source: https://archive.org/details/chronicdiseaseoohahn, retrieved December 13, 2019).

Hauser, Andrea. *What is Homeopathic Medicine?*, http://hauserhomeopathy.com/what-is-homeopathy.html (retrieved March 1, 2019).

Hilarius-Ford, Anne. *Origins and development of Facial Reflexology*. https://www.energyreflexology.com.au/origins-and-development-of-facial-reflexology (retrieved December 13, 2019).

Homeopathy Plus, *The Vital Force*. http://homeopathyplus.com/tutorial-7-the-vital-force/, (retrieved December 5, 2019).

Jensen, Bernard, Bodeen, Donald. *Visions of Health. Understanding Iridology*. New York: Avery, 1992.

Iyengar, B.K.S. *Light on Pranayama*. London: Unwin, 1983.

———. *Yoga: The Path to Holistic Health*. London: Dorling Kindersley, 2008.

Jwing-Ming, Yang. *The Essence of Tai Chi Chi Kung*. Jamaica Plain, MA: YMAA Publication Center, 1990.

Keet, Louise. *The Reflexology Bible*. London: Octopus, 2008.

Kent, James Tyler. *Lectures on Homeopathic Philosophy*. Chicago: Ehrhart & Karl, 1919 (online source: https://archive.org/details/lecturesonhomoeookentgoog, retrieved December 13, 2019).

Knipschild, P. "Looking for gall bladder disease in the patient's iris." *British Medical Journal* 297, (December 17, 1988) 1578-81.

Koehler, Gerhard. *The Handbook of Homeopathy. Its Principles and Practice*. Rochester: Healing Arts, 1989.

Kretsinger, Robert. *History and Philosophy of Biology*. Hackensack, NJ: World Scientific Publishing Company, 2015.

Krieger, Dolores. *The Personal Practice of Therapeutic Touch*. Santa Fe: Bear & Co, 1993.

Kunz, Barbara & Kevin. *Complete Reflexology for Life*. New York: DK, 2007.

Kushi, Michio. *Natural Healing through Macrobiotics*. Tokyo: Japan Publications, 1978.

———. *The Book of Macrobiotics: The Universal Way of Health and Happiness*. Tokyo: Japan Publications, 1977.

Bibliography

———. *Your Face Never Lies*. Wayne, NJ: Avery, 1983.
Kushi, Michio, and Jannetta, Phillip. *Macrobiotics and Oriental Medicine: An Introduction to Holistic Health*, Tokyo: Japan Publications, 1991.
Kushi, Michio, and Oredson, Olivia. *Macrobiotic Palm Healing, Energy at Your Fingertips*, Tokyo: Japan Publications, 1988.
Lad, Vasant. *Ayurveda, The Science of Self-Healing*. Wilmot, WI: Lotus, 1984.
———. *The Complete Book of Ayurvedic Home Remedies*. London: Piatkus, 1999.
Liao, Waysun. *T'ai Chi Classics*. Boston: Shambhala, 1990.
Lübeck, Walter. *The Complete Reiki Handbook: Basic Introduction and Methods of Natural Application*. Twin Lakes, WI: Lotus Press, 2009.
Lübeck, Walter, et al. *The Spirit of Reiki: The Complete Handbook of the Reiki System*. Twin Lakes, WI: Lotus, 2001.
Mahadevan, T.M.P. *Invitation to Indian Philosophy*. New Delhi: Arnold – Heinemann, 1974.
Mahesh, Maharishi. *Beacon Light Of The Himalayas*. 1955. http://www.paulmason.info/gurudev/Beacon.htm (retrieved March 1, 2019).
———. *The Science of Being and the Art of Living*. New York: New American Library, 1968.
Maoshing Ni (translator). *The Yellow Emperor's Classic of Medicine: A New Translation of the Neijing Suwen with Commentary*. Boston: Shambhala, 2011.
Master, Farokh J. et al., *Bach Flower Remedies for Everyone*. New Delhi: Jain Publishers, 1994.
McCall, Timothy. *Yoga as Medicine: The Yogic Prescription for Health and Healing*. New York: Bantam, 2007.
Mediks Ltd, "How does SU JOK heal," online source: https://www.mediks-bg.com/how-does-su-jok-heal (retrieved December 12, 2019).
Michio Kushi, Phillip Jannetta. *Macrobiotics and Oriental Medicine*. Tokyo: Japan Publications, 1991.
Mole, Peter. *Acupuncture: Energy Balancing for Body, Mind & Spirit*. Shaftesbury, UK: Element, 1998.
Mookerjee, Ajit. *Kundalini: The Arousal of the Inner Energy*. Rochester: Destiny, 1986.
Morant, Georges Soulié de. *Chinese Acupuncture*. Brookline, MA: Paradigm, 1996.
Münstedt, K., et al. "Can iridology detect susceptibility to cancer? A prospective case-controlled study." *Journal of Alternative and Complementary Medicine* 11,3 (June 11, 2005) 515–9.
O'Mathuna, Donal, and Larimore, Walt, *Alternative Medicine: The Christian Handbook*, Grand Rapids, MI: Zondervan, 2001.
Patanjali. *Yoga Sutra*. New York: Penguin, 2008.
Pfeifer, Samuel. *Healing at Any Price?, The Hidden Dangers of Alternative Medicine*. Milton Keynes, UK: Word, 1988.
Plato. *Euthyphro, Apology, Crito, Phaedo, Phaedrus*. Harvard: Harvard University Press, 1914 (reprinted 2005).
Radhakrishnan, Sarvepalli. *The Principal Upanishads*. London: George Allen & Unwin, 1968.
Rand, William Lee. *Reiki for a New Millennium*. Southfield, MI: Vision, 1998.
Rosenthal, Stan (translator). *The Tao Te Ching*. http://enlight.lib.ntu.edu.tw/FULLTEXT/JR-AN/an142304.pdf (retrieved December 13, 2019).
Sanchez, Camilo. *Daoist Meridian Yoga*. London: Singing Dragon, 2016.

Bibliography

Schnorrenberger, Claus C. *Chen-Chiu: The Original Acupuncture*. Boston: Wisdom, 2003.

Singh, Simon, and Edzard, Ernst. *Trick or Treatment? Alternative Medicine on Trial*. London: Bantam, 2008.

Sivananda, Swami. *Concentration and Meditation*. Shivanandanagar: Divine Life Society, 1983.

———. *The Practice of Yoga*. Shivanandanagar: Divine Life Society, 2006.

Shiva-Samhita. Translator: Rai Bahadur Srisa Chandra Vasu, online source: https://archive.org/stream/SivaSamhita/SivaSamhita_djvu.txt (retrieved December 13, 2019).

Sponzili, Osvaldo. *Iniziazione all'Iridologia: Diagnosi e terapia mediante l'osservazione dell'iride* [*Initiation in Iridology: Diagnosis and Therapy by Observing the Iris*]. Roma: Edizioni Mediterranee, 2000.

Steiner, Rudolf. *An Esoteric Cosmology*, part V, "Yoga in East and West," Paris, 1906, Schmidt Number: S-1325, online source: https://wn.rsarchive.org/Lectures/GA094/English/SGP1978/19060529p01.html (retrieved December 13, 2019).

———. "Cosmic Ego and Human Ego. The Nature of Christ the Resurrected," Munich, January 9,1912, Schmidt Number: S-2518, online source: http://wn.rsarchive.org/Lectures/CosEgo_index.html (retrieved December 13, 2019).

———. "Karma of the Higher Beings," Hamburg, May 25, 1910, Schmidt Number: S-2237, online source: https://wn.rsarchive.org/Lectures/GA120/English/RSP1984/19100525p01.html (retrieved December 13, 2019).

———. *Medicine, An Introductory Reader*. Forest Row: Sophia, 2003.

Steiner, Rudolf, and Wegman, Ita. *Fundamentals of Therapy: An Extension of the Art of Healing through Spiritual Knowledge*. London: Rudolf Steiner Press, 1983.

Stenger, Victor. "Quantum Quackery." *Skeptical Inquirer* 21.1 (January / February 1997) 37–40.

———. *Physics and Psychics: The Search for a World Beyond the Senses*. Buffalo, NY: Prometheus, 1990.

Stewart, Gary P., et al. *Basic Questions on Alternative Medicine: What Is Good and What Is Not?* Grand Rapids: Kregel, 1998.

Svatmarama. *The Hathayogapradipika*. London: Aquarian, 1992.

The Tao Te Ching, translator Stan Rosenthal, online source: http://enlight.lib.ntu.edu.tw/FULLTEXT/JR-AN/an142304.pdf (retrieved December 13, 2019).

Turgeon, Madeleine. *Découvrons la réflexologie-Technique d'acupuncture sans aiguilles*, [*Discovering Reflexology. Acupuncture technique without needles*]. Boucherville, Quebec: Mortagne, 1990.

———. *Energie et réflexologie - La polarité à votre portée* [*Energy and reflexology - the polarity at your fingertips*]. Boucherville, Quebec: Mortagne, 1985.

Tyler, Gina. *Homeopathy and Radiaesthesia*. online source: http://hpathy.com/homeopathy-papers/homeopathy-and-radiaesthesia/2/, (retrieved December 13, 2019).

USCCB, Committee on Doctrine. *Guidelines for Evaluating Reiki as an Alternative Therapy*. March 3, 2009. http://www.usccb.org/_cs_upload/8092_1.pdf (retrieved December 13, 2019).

———. *The Catechism of the Catholic Church* for the United States of America, Washington, 1994

Bibliography

Usui, Mikao, and Petter, Frank Arjava. *The Original Reiki Handbook of Dr. Mikao Usui: The Traditional Usui Reiki Ryoho Treatment Positions and Numerous Reiki Techniques for Health and Well-being*. Twin Lakes, WI: Lotus, 2000.

Vennells, David F. *Reflexology for Beginners: Healing through Foot Massage of Pressure Points*. St. Paul, MN: Llewellyn, 2001.

Vithoulkas, George. *Homeopathy: Medicine for the New Millennium*. Alonissos, Greece: International Academy of Classical Homeopathy, 2000.

———. *The Science of Homeopathy*. New Delhi: Jain Publishers, 1986.

Vivekananda, Swami. *Lectures on Raja Yoga*. London: Longman, Green & Co, 1896.

Watkins, Arleen, Bickel, William. "A Study of the Kirlian Effect." *The Skeptical Inquirer* 10, 3 (1986) 244–257.

Wills, Pauline. *Reflexology and Colour Therapy*. Dorset, UK: Element, 1998.

Index

Acupuncture, ix, 41n9, 54, 58, 60–61, 70, 72, 75–88, 93, 117, 118n49, 130
angels, 4–5, 7, 21, 37, 56, 60, 62–64, 67, 69–70, 87, 130
Anthroposophical medicine, ix, 27–38, 130
asana, 16–17, 20, 23, 47–48, 75
astral body, 29–34, 58, 95
auricular reflexology, 88, 91–92
Ayurveda, ix, 21, 26, 39–51, 57, 79, 102, 126, 130, 133

Bach floral remedies, ix, 97n39, 124–28, 130
Buddhism, Buddhist 16, 53–54, 56, 62–65, 75, 91, 97–100

chakra, 9, 18–23, 55–57, 60, 68, 70, 75n7, 95–96
Chi, 53–54, 58, 74n5, 75–80, 82, 84, 86–87, 91–94, 97–98, 117, 118n49, 130–31, 133
Chinese Medicine, 69, 72, 75–79, 81, 83, 86, 92, 94n20

Dien Chan, 91–92
dosha, 39–43, 47–48
dualism, 1–3, 5–6

etheric body, 6, 29–30, 32–35, 38n40, 58–59, 95, 114, 120

fundamental elements, 31, 35, 40, 78, 82–84

Hatha Yoga, 14–19, 21, 47–48, 55, 75n7, 96
Hinduism, 2, 5–6, 9–10, 12, 15–17, 20–24, 26, 28–29, 31, 40, 43–47, 49–51, 54–56, 60, 62–64, 67, 69–70, 72–75, 77, 95–96, 98, 102, 125, 130
homeopathy, ix, 101, 103–13, 116–21, 123–26, 130–31
hylomorphism, 3

I Ching, 91, 94
initiation, 19, 39n3, 44–45, 54, 60, 62, 66–67, 69, 75, 131
iridology, ix, 101–2

karma, 9, 11, 13, 23–26, 28–29, 38, 44, 51–52, 56–57, 67, 95, 98–100, 102, 130
Kirlian effect, 56n21, 58–59, 93n15
kundalini, 9, 15, 17–21, 23, 55, 96

macrobiotics, ix, 68–71
mantra, 19–20, 22, 45–48, 62–63, 70, 96
massage, 51, 85, 89–91, 93n15, 96–97
meditation, 13n11, 14–16, 18, 20–23, 43–48, 51, 61–62, 67–68, 70, 75–76, 130
meridian, 58, 70, 74, 77, 79–82, 88, 93n15
mesmerism, 116–18
miasm, 109–10, 121, 123–24
moxibustion, 80, 85

nadi, 17–18, 48, 95

Index

original sin, 121–23

pantheism, pantheistic, 9–10, 13, 15, 44–45, 49–50, 69–70, 72
physicalism, 1–5
placebo, viii, 85n36, 92, 103–4, 117, 124
potency, 107, 109, 112n29
prana, 9, 12, 17–19, 22–23, 48, 54, 58, 77, 95, 131, 133
pranayama, 17–18, 48
pressopuncture, 88
psora, 109–11, 118, 121–22, 124
pulse, 41, 49, 70, 79, 82, 85–86, 108

Qigong, 53, 60, 74–76

reflex zones, 88–93, 96–97
reflexology, ix, 54, 61, 70, 88–93, 95–98, 100, 130
Reiki, ix, 20–22, 53–70, 93n15, 94–95, 97n39, 100, 117–18, 126, 130, 133
reincarnation, 2, 9, 11, 13, 23–26, 28, 32, 38, 44, 51, 56, 67, 96, 98, 100, 102, 130
resurrection, 5, 25, 66, 134

Shamanism, 55
shen, 78
Siddha Yoga, 19–20, 60
Su Jok, 91–92
succussion, 106, 115–16
sushumna, 17–19, 48, 70, 96

Tai Chi, 74–76
Taoism, 54–55, 69–70, 72–74, 83–84, 89, 91–92, 94
Therapeutic Touch, ix, 68–70
Transcendental Meditation, 43–45, 62

vital force, 64, 70, 75n8, 113–21, 124

water-memory effect, 112

yin and *yang*, 70–71, 73–77, 79, 93
Yoga (see also Hatha Yoga and Siddha Yoga), ix, 9, 13–23, 43, 46–47, 48n49, 51, 60, 62, 63n55, 74–76, 130

www.ingramcontent.com/pod-product-compliance
Lightning Source LLC
Chambersburg PA
CBHW072147160426
43197CB00012B/2277